JUICING FOR CANCER PATIENTS

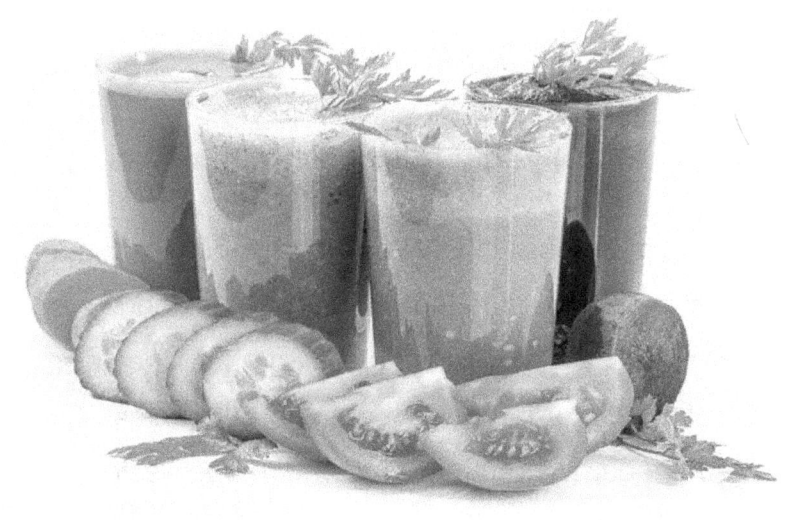

The ultimate guide to using nature to heal cancer

Kelly k. Kerr

Table of Contents

Cancer is a complex group of diseases characterized by the uncontrolled growth and spread of abnormal cells. While the causes of cancer are multifactorial, there is growing interest in the role of hydration and detoxification in cancer prevention and management. This comprehensive guide explores the relationship between hydration, detoxification, and cancer, shedding light on how these factors can impact cancer risk, treatment, and overall well-being.

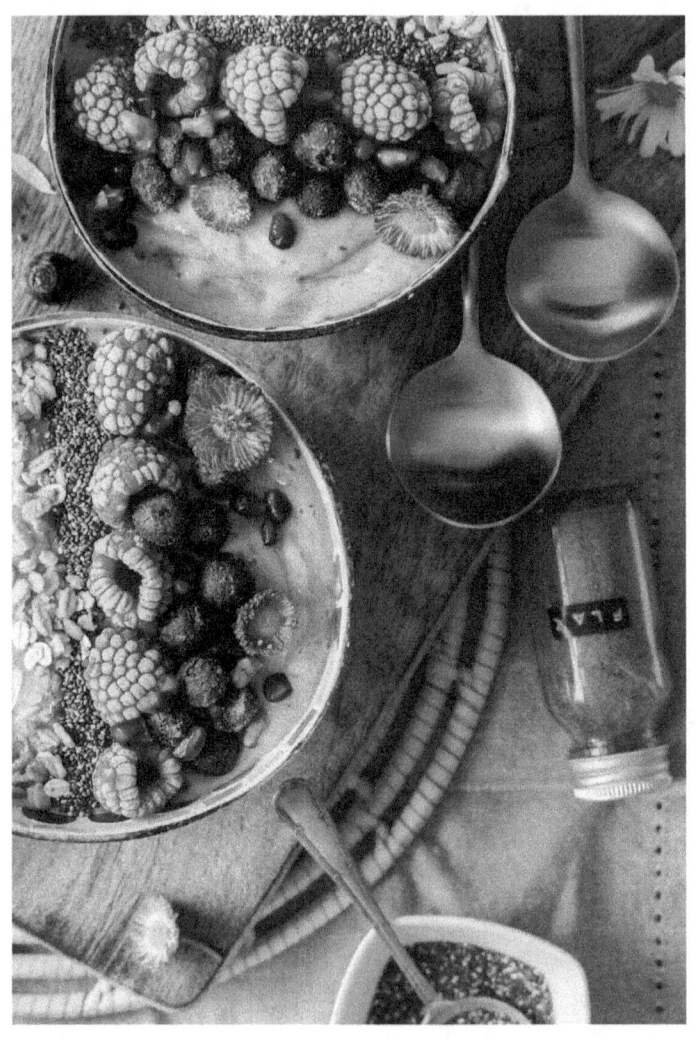

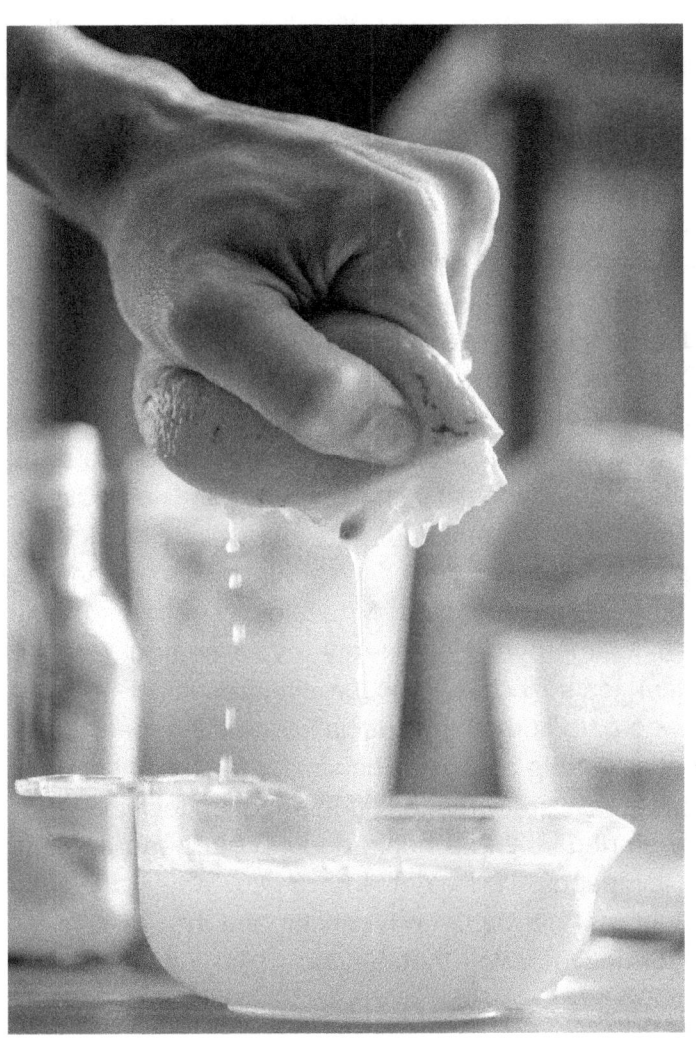

Introduction

Emily had battled cancer for years, enduring countless treatments and surgeries. But one day, a serendipitous encounter changed her life forever.

While waiting for her chemotherapy session at the local hospital, Emily struck up a conversation with a fellow patient named Sarah. They shared their stories of struggle and hope, and Sarah mentioned a book she had been reading about the potential healing powers of natural juices. Intrigued, Emily decided to give it a try.Over the next few months, Emily immersed herself in research about the benefits of fresh, organic juices. She began experimenting with various combinations of fruits and vegetables, seeking the perfect blend to boost her immune system and promote healing. Her kitchen became a laboratory, filled with vibrant colors and the soothing hum of juicers Miraculously, Emily's health began to improve. Her energy levels soared, and her medical tests showed encouraging results. She knew she was onto something special, something that had the potential to help others facing similar battles. Inspired by her progress, Emily made a life-changing decision.

Emily started writing a book, pouring her heart and soul into its pages. She detailed her journey, the ups, anddowns of her battle with cancer, and the

transformative role that juices had played in her recovery.

Chapter1: Cancer and Nutrition

Cancer is a complex group of diseases characterized by the uncontrolled growth and spread of abnormal cells in the body. While genetics and environmental factors play significant roles in cancer development, emerging research has shown that nutrition can also have a profound impact on cancer risk, prevention, and treatment.

Cancer and Nutrition: The Connection

Cancer Prevention

A diet rich in fruits and vegetables, whole grains, and legumes provides essential vitamins, minerals, and antioxidants that help protect cells from damage and reduce the risk of cancer.

Consuming a variety of colorful fruits and vegetables can provide a wide range of phytochemicals, which have been shown to have cancer-fighting properties.

Limiting the consumption of processed foods, sugary beverages, and red and processed meats can lower the risk of cancer.

Maintaining a Healthy Weight

Obesity is a significant risk factor for many types of cancer, including breast, colon, and pancreatic cancer. Proper nutrition and portion control are crucial for maintaining a healthy weight, reducing cancer risk.

Nutrition During Cancer Treatment

Cancer treatments like chemotherapy and radiation therapy can have side effects that affect appetite and nutrient absorption. It's essential to work with a healthcare team to develop a personalized nutrition plan.

High-protein diets can help in repairing tissues damaged during treatment, while avoiding certain foods that may interact negatively with treatments is important.

Managing Side Effects

Nutritional strategies can help manage common cancer treatment side effects like nausea, diarrhea, and mouth sores.

Small, frequent meals, bland foods, and staying hydrated can alleviate digestive issues.

Choosing soft, easy-to-swallow foods can help with mouth sores and difficulty swallowing.

Special Dietary Considerations

Some cancer patients may require specialized diets due to specific treatments or conditions. For example, a low-fiber diet may be recommended for those with bowel obstructions.

Registered dietitians can provide individualized guidance to address these needs.

Nutritional Supplements

While whole foods are generally the best source of nutrients, some cancer patients may benefit from supplements under medical supervision.
Common supplements include vitamin D, calcium, and omega-3 fatty acids, but their use should be discussed with a healthcare provider.

Types and Stages of Cancer

There are numerous types of cancer, each with its unique characteristics, risk factors, and treatment approaches. Additionally, cancer typically progresses through stages, which indicate the extent of the disease and help determine the most appropriate treatment. In this comprehensive content, we will explore the various types of cancer and the stages of cancer progression.

Types of Cancer

Carcinomas :Carcinomas are the most common type of cancer and originate in the epithelial tissues that cover the body's surfaces and line organs and glands. They are further categorized into subtypes:

Adenocarcinoma: Arising in glands that produce mucus, such as the lung, prostate, breast, and colon.

Squamous cell carcinoma: Developing in the squamous cells that form the skin's outer layer or line the respiratory and digestive tracts.

Basal cell carcinoma: Usually occurring in the basal cells at the bottom of the epidermis, primarily on sun-exposed skin.

Sarcomas :Sarcomas develop in the body's connective tissues, including bones, muscles, tendons, and cartilage. They are less common than carcinomas and include osteosarcoma (bone), liposarcoma (fat), and leiomyosarcoma (smooth muscle).

Leukemias

Leukemias are cancers of the blood and bone marrow, where blood-forming cells become abnormal and crowd out healthy blood cells. The four main types are acute lymphoblastic leukemia (ALL), acute myeloid leukemia (AML), chronic lymphocytic leukemia (CLL), and chronic myeloid leukemia (CML).

Lymphomas

Lymphomas affect the lymphatic system, which includes lymph nodes, spleen, and bone marrow. The two primary categories are Hodgkin lymphoma and non-Hodgkin lymphoma (NHL).

Myelomas

Myelomas form in plasma cells, a type of white blood cell responsible for producing antibodies. Multiple myeloma is the most common form of this cancer.

Central Nervous System (CNS) Cancers

These cancers affect the brain and spinal cord. Gliomas, meningiomas, and medulloblastomas are some examples.

Germ Cell Tumors

Germ cell tumors develop in the cells that give rise to sperm or eggs. They most often occur in the testes or ovaries.

Neuroendocrine Tumors

These tumors arise in cells that release hormones into the bloodstream and can occur in various organs, including the pancreas, lungs, and gastrointestinal tract.

Stages of Cancer Progression

Cancer stages describe the extent and severity of the disease, aiding in treatment decisions and prognosis assessment. The most common system for staging cancer is the TNM system:

1. Tumor (T)

This category describes the size and extent of the primary tumor. T stages range from 0 (in situ, localized) to T4 (extensive local growth or invasion into nearby structures).

2. Lymph Nodes (N)

N stages indicate whether cancer has spread to nearby lymph nodes. N0 means no lymph node involvement, while N3 signifies extensive lymph node involvement.

3. Metastasis (M)

The M stage indicates whether cancer has spread to distant organs or tissues. M0 means no distant metastasis, while M1 denotes the presence of metastatic cancer.

Combining the T, N, and M stages yields an overall cancer stage, usually expressed as stages 0 (in situ) to IV (advanced disease). The higher the stage, the more extensive the cancer.

In addition to TNM staging, cancer stages are often categorized into broader groups:

Stage 0: In situ cancers, where abnormal cells are confined to their place of origin.

Stage I and II: Early-stage cancers, typically smaller in size and less invasive.

Stage III: Locally advanced cancers with extensive lymph node involvement.

Stage IV: Advanced cancers that have spread to distant parts of the body.

Understanding the type noand stage of cancer is crucial for healthcare professionals to determine the most appropriate treatment plan, predict prognosis, and assess the overall impact on a patient's health.

It's important to note that this content provides a general overview of cancer types and staging. Each specific cancer type may have its unique features, risk factors, and treatment options, and individuals should consult with healthcare professionals for personalized information and guidance. Regular screenings and early detection remain essential in improving cancer outcomes, underscoring the importance of cancer awareness and prevention.

How Cancer Affects Nutrition

Cancer can impact nutrition in several ways.

Appetite changes: Cancer and its treatments can lead to loss of appetite, making it difficult to consume enough calories and nutrients.

Weight loss: Unintentional weight loss is common in cancer patients, which can result in muscle wasting and weakness.

Malabsorption: Some cancers and notreatments can interfere with the body's ability to absorb nutrients from food.

Nutrient deficiencies: Cancer patients may develop deficiencies in essential nutrients like vitamins, minerals, and proteins, affecting overall health.

Digestive problems: Cancer-related gastrointestinal issues can cause nausea, vomiting, diarrhea, and difficulty swallowing, making it challenging to maintain a balanced diet.

Changes in taste and smell: Altered taste and smell perceptions can affect food preferences and make certain foods less appealing.

Nutritional support: Many cancer patients require nutritional support, such as dietary counseling, supplements, or even tube feeding, to meet their nutritional needs.

Immune system suppression: Malnutrition in cancer patients can weaken the immune system, potentially impacting the ability to fight the disease.

Managing nutrition during cancer treatment often involves personalized dietary plans and support from healthcare professionals to maintain strength and overall well-being

Nutritional Needs During Cancer Treatment

Nutritional needs during cancer treatments are of paramount importance, as they play a crucial role in supporting the body's ability to cope with the disease and its therapies. Cancer treatments, such as chemotherapy, radiation therapy, and surgery, can place significant demands on the body, affecting appetite, digestion, and nutrient absorption. Addressing these needs can help manage treatment-related side effects, maintain overall health, and improve the chances of a successful outcome. Here's a comprehensive overview of the nutritional needs during cancer treatments:

Adequate Calories: Cancer treatments can increase the body's energy requirements. Patients often need more calories to maintain their weight and energy levels. Choosing nutrient-dense foods, such as whole grains, lean proteins, and healthy fats, can provide the necessary calories while supporting overall health.

Protein: Protein is essential for tissue repair and immune function. Patients undergoing cancer treatment should aim to include lean sources of protein, such as poultry, fish, beans, and tofu, in their diet.

Hydration: Maintaining proper hydration is crucial, especially if treatment-related side effects like vomiting or diarrhea are present. Drinking enough fluids helps prevent dehydration and supports various bodily functions.

Vitamins and Minerals: Certain vitamins and minerals, including vitamin D, calcium, and magnesium, are important for bone health. Chemotherapy and steroids can affect bone density, so it's vital to ensure an adequate intake of these nutrients.

Fiber: Adequate dietary fiber can help prevent constipation, a common side effect of some cancer treatments. Fiber-rich foods like fruits, vegetables, and whole grains should be included in the diet.

Antioxidants: Antioxidant-rich foods, such as berries, dark leafy greens, and colorful vegetables, can help protect cells from damage caused by cancer treatments and may support the body's natural defense mechanisms.

Omega-3 Fatty Acids: These healthy fats, found in fish, flaxseeds, and walnuts, may have anti-inflammatory properties and can support heart and brain health during cancer treatment.

Small, Frequent Meals: Eating smaller, more frequent meals can help manage nausea and maintain energy levels, particularly if appetite is reduced.

Supplements: In some cases, healthcare providers may recommend specific supplements, such as iron, vitamin B12, or folic acid, if deficiencies are identified through blood tests.

Individualized Plans: Nutritional needs can vary widely among cancer patients, so it's essential to work with a registered dietitian or nutritionist to create a personalized nutrition plan. They can assess individual needs, monitor weight changes, and adjust the diet accordingly.

Monitor for Food Safety: Cancer treatments can weaken the immune system, making patients more susceptible to infections. It's crucial to practice food safety measures, like washing hands and thoroughly cooking food, to reduce the risk of foodborne illnesses.

Emotional Support: Coping with cancer and its treatments can be emotionally challenging. Emotional well-being is closely tied to nutrition. Support groups or counseling may help patients maintain a positive attitude toward food and eating.

In conclusion, meeting nutritional needs during cancer treatments is a vital aspect of overall care. A well-balanced diet can help manage treatment-related side effects, maintain strength, and support the body's healing process. Collaboration with healthcare providers and registered dietitians is essential to tailor dietary recommendations to individual circumstances, ensuring the best possible outcomes for cancer patients.

Chapter2: Juicing Basics

Juicing can be a helpful addition to the diet of someone with cancer, but it's important to approach it carefully. Here are some juicing basics for cancer:

Consult with a healthcare professional: Before making any dietary changes, including juicing, it's crucial to consult with your healthcare team. They can provide personalized advice based on your specific cancer type, treatment, and nutritional needs.

Choose the right ingredients: Opt for fresh, organic fruits and vegetables that are rich in vitamins, minerals, and antioxidants. Dark leafy greens, carrots, beets, berries, and citrus fruits are good choices.

Avoid sugary or processed ingredients: Stay away from high-sugar fruits and processed juices, as excess sugar can feed cancer cells and weaken the immune system.

Balance your juices: Aim for a balance of fruits and vegetables in your juices to provide a variety of nutrients. Vegetables should make up the majority of your juice.

Include ginger and turmeric: Both ginger and turmeric have anti-inflammatory properties and may be beneficial for cancer patients. Add small amounts to your juices for flavor and potential health benefits.

Go easy on quantity: Don't overdo it with juicing. Small, frequent servings are often better tolerated than large quantities at once.

Drink immediately: Freshly made juices are most nutritious when consumed immediately. If you can't drink them right away, store them in an airtight container in the refrigerator for a short period.

Monitor your tolerance: Some cancer patients may experience digestive issues or sensitivities to certain ingredients. Pay attention to how your body reacts and adjust your recipes accordingly.

Hydrate with water: Remember that juicing should complement your overall hydration, not replace it. Drink plenty of water throughout the day.

Use juicing as a supplement: Juicing should be part of a well-balanced diet and not the sole source of nutrition. Ensure you're getting a variety of foods to meet your nutritional needs.

Remember that while juicing can provide valuable nutrients, it should be integrated into a holistic approach to cancer care, including medical treatments and a balanced diet. Always follow your healthcare provider's recommendations for managing cancer through nutrition.

Getting Started with Juicing

Cancer is a formidable adversary, but a well-balanced diet can be a crucial ally in the fight against this disease. Juicing is gaining popularity as a nutritious and flavorful way to supplement cancer treatment and boost overall health. In this comprehensive guide, we'll explore the benefits of juicing for cancer, the best ingredients to use, and some tips to get you started on your juicing journey.

Section 1: Understanding the Role of Juicing in Cancer Care

The Power of Nutrition:Proper nutrition plays a pivotal role in cancer treatment and recovery. Juicing provides a concentrated source of essential vitamins, minerals, and antioxidants that can support your body's healing processes.
Nutritional Goals: Identify your specific nutritional needs based on your cancer type, treatment plan, and overall health. Consult with a healthcare professional or registered dietitian to create a tailored juicing plan.

Section 2: Choosing the Right Ingredients

Cancer-Fighting Fruits: Incorporate fruits like berries, citrus, and kiwi rich in antioxidants, vitamins, and immune-boosting properties.
Leafy Greens: Dark leafy greens such as kale, spinach, and Swiss chard are packed with nutrients like folate and chlorophyll, which may help fight cancer.

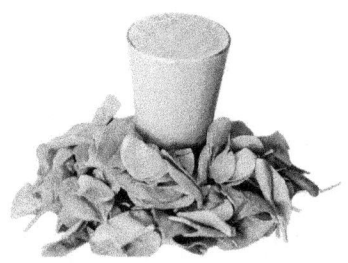

Cruciferous Vegetables:Broccoli, cauliflower, and cabbage contain compounds that have been linked to cancer prevention.

Turmeric and Ginger:These spices possess anti-inflammatory properties that can be beneficial during cancer treatment.

Section 3 Juicing Equipment and Techniques

Choosing a Juicer:Explore the different types of juicers, such as centrifugal, masticating, and cold-press, to find the one that suits your needs and budget.

Preparing Ingredients:Wash and chop fruits and vegetables before juicing. Remove any inedible parts and seeds.

Mixing Recipes:Experiment with various combinations to find flavors you enjoy while ensuring you meet your nutritional goals.

Section 4: Safety Considerations

Organic Produce:Whenever possible, choose organic produce to minimize exposure to pesticides and chemicals.
Hygiene:Maintain proper hygiene by cleaning your juicer thoroughly after each use to prevent contamination.
Portion Control:Be mindful of portion sizes to avoid excessive calorie intake.

Section 5: Integrating Juicing into Your Cancer Care Plan

Consult Your Healthcare Team:Discuss your juicing plan with your oncologist or healthcare provider to ensure it complements your treatment.
Monitor Your Body:Pay attention to how your body responds to juicing. Make adjustments as needed to address any adverse effects or allergies.
Emotional Well-being:Juicing can be a enjoyable and therapeutic part of your cancer journey. Savor the flavors and use it as a way to relax and nourish both your body and mind.

Choosing the Right Juicer

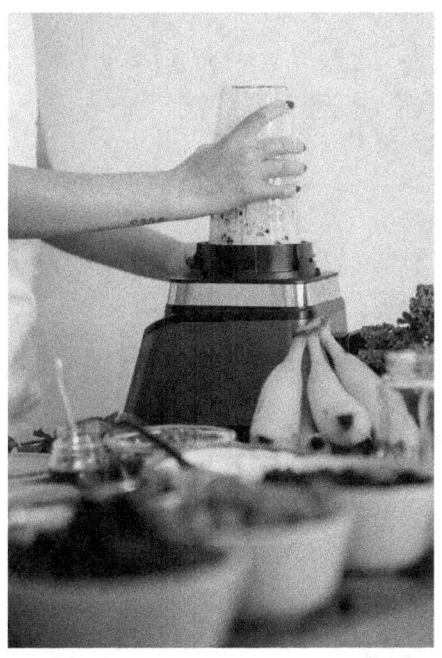

Cancer patients often face unique dietary challenges, and maintaining proper nutrition is crucial during their treatment journey. One way to support their nutritional needs is through juicing fresh fruits and vegetables. However, choosing the right juicer is essential to ensure that the juices provide maximum benefits while minimizing potential risks. In this comprehensive guide, we will explore the factors to consider when selecting a juicer for cancer patients.

Types of Juicers:
There are several types of juicers available on the market, each with its own advantages and disadvantages. Understanding these options is essential when choosing the right juicer for cancer patients.

Centrifugal Juicers: These juicers work by rapidly spinning the produce and using centrifugal force to extract juice. They are generally less expensive and quick but may generate some heat, potentially reducing the nutritional value of the juice over time.

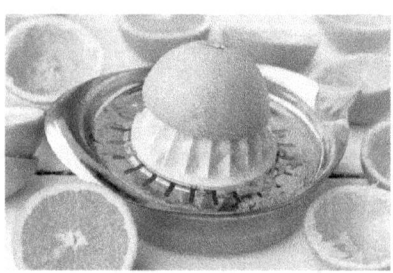

Masticating Juicers (Cold Press Juicers):
Masticating juicers use a slower, crushing action to extract juice. They tend to preserve more nutrients and enzymes, making them a preferred choice for

cancer patients.

Triturating Juicers (Twin Gear Juicers): These juicers have two gears that rotate slowly to extract juice. They are known for producing the highest quality juice with minimal nutrient loss but can be more expensive and complex to use.

Nutrient Preservation: For cancer patients, it's crucial to retain as many nutrients as possible in the juice. Masticating and triturating juicers are better at preserving essential vitamins, minerals, and enzymes compared to centrifugal juicers.

Ease of Use: Consider the patient's condition and physical abilities. Some juicers are easier to operate and clean than others. Look for models with user-friendly features like wide chutes for easy feeding and dishwasher-safe parts for convenience.

Yield: Cancer patients may need to consume larger quantities of juice to meet their nutritional needs. Choose a juicer that provides a high juice yield, as this can help reduce food waste and save money in the long run.

Noise Level: Cancer treatment can be physically and emotionally taxing. Opt for a juicer with a quieter operation to avoid causing unnecessary stress or discomfort to the patient.

Budget: Juicers come in a wide price range. While it's essential to consider the patient's budget, it's also important to balance this with the juicer's performance and durability. Investing in a quality juicer can be a worthwhile long-term decision.

Cleaning and Maintenance: Cancer patients may have limited energy and mobility. Choose a juicer that is easy to clean and maintain, as this can make the juicing process more manageable for them

Safety Features: Look for juicers with safety features like overload protection and secure locking mechanisms to reduce the risk of accidents, especially when patients may be fatigued or weak.

Warranty and Customer Support: Check the warranty and availability of customer support for the chosen juicer. A reliable warranty and responsive customer service can provide peace of mind in case of any issues.

Selecting High-Quality Produce

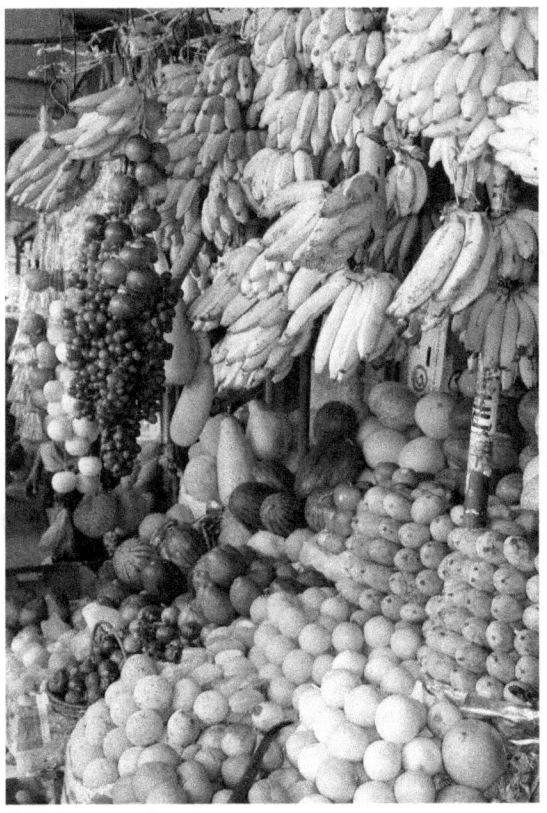

The link between diet and cancer risk has been extensively studied, and it's widely recognized that the foods we consume can either promote or protect against cancer. Fruits, in particular, play a crucial role in cancer prevention due to their rich content of vitamins, minerals, fiber, and antioxidants. However, the quality of the produce you choose can significantly impact its cancer-fighting potential. In this comprehensive guide, we will explore how to select high-quality fruits to reduce the risk of cancer and promote overall health.

Organic vs. Conventional: Organic produce is grown without synthetic pesticides and genetically modified organisms (GMOs), which may have uncertain long-term health effects.

While organic fruits are ideal, conventional options can still be nutritious and low in cancer risk when properly washed and prepared.

Colorful Variety: Aim for a diverse selection of fruits with vibrant colors, as different pigments indicate various antioxidants and phytochemicals beneficial for cancer prevention.Examples of colorful cancer-fighting fruits include berries (blueberries, strawberries, raspberries), oranges, and dark leafy greens (kale, spinach).

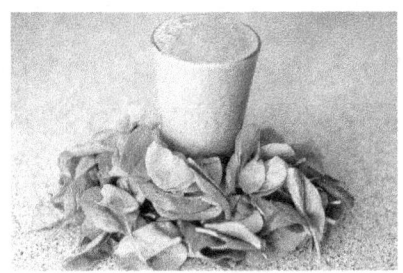

Freshness Matters: Fresh fruits generally contain higher nutrient levels than those that have been stored for extended periods.Shop at local farmers' markets when possible to access fresher produce that hasn't traveled long distances.

Check for Ripeness: Choose fruits that are ripe and ready to eat to ensure optimal taste and nutrient content.Avoid overripe fruits, which may have higher sugar content and lower nutritional value.

Seasonal Choices: Opt for seasonal fruits as they are more likely to be fresh, locally sourced, and cost-effective.Seasonal fruits also offer variety throughout the year.

Pesticide Residue: Refer to the Environmental Working Group's (EWG) "Dirty Dozen" and "Clean Fifteen" lists to prioritize organic options for produce that tends to have higher pesticide residue.Washing fruits thoroughly can help reduce pesticide residues on conventionally grown produce.

Fiber-Rich Picks: Choose fruits that are rich in dietary fiber, as fiber can aid in digestion and reduce the risk of colorectal cancer.Examples include apples, pears, and citrus fruits.

Whole vs. Processed: Whole fruits are preferable to fruit juices and processed snacks, as they contain more fiber and fewer added sugars.Processed fruit products may lack the cancer-fighting benefits of fresh, whole fruits.

Storage and Handling: Store fruits properly to maintain their freshness and nutritional value.Follow guidelines for refrigeration and use within a reasonable timeframe.

Individual Preferences: Consider personal preferences, allergies, and dietary restrictions when choosing fruits to ensure a balanced and enjoyable diet.

Proper Juicing Techniques

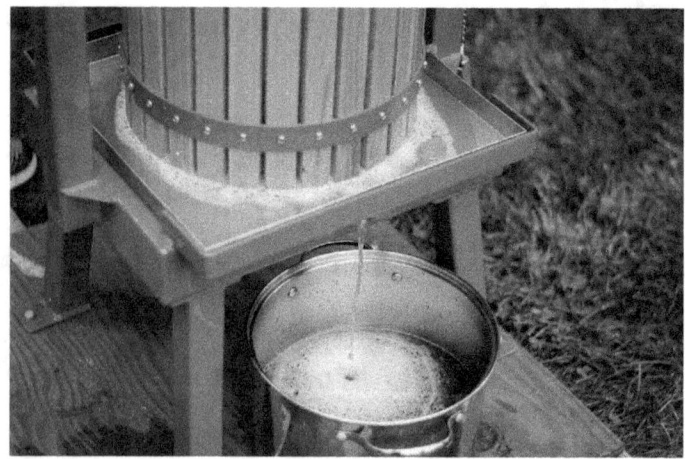

Juicing can be a part of a healthy diet, but it's important to approach it with caution, especially in relation to cancer. Here are some proper juicing techniques to consider:

Consult a Healthcare Professional: If you or someone you know is dealing with cancer, it's crucial to consult with a healthcare professional or

a registered dietitian before making significant dietary changes, including juicing.

Choose the Right Ingredients: Select fruits and vegetables that are rich in antioxidants, vitamins, and minerals, which can support overall health. Examples include leafy greens, carrots, beets, berries, and citrus fruits.

Organic Produce: Opt for organic produce when possible to reduce exposure to pesticides and chemicals.

Avoid Excessive Sugar: Limit fruits that are high in sugar, as cancer cells can feed on sugar.

Consider using more vegetables than fruits in your juices.

Variety is Key: Rotate your ingredients to ensure a diverse range of nutrients in your diet. Different fruits and vegetables offer unique health benefits.

Fresh and Clean: Wash your produce thoroughly to remove any contaminants. Use a clean juicer to avoid bacterial contamination.

Moderation: Don't rely solely on juicing as your primary source of nutrition. It's best used as a supplement to a balanced diet.

Avoid Fasting: Fasting or extreme juicing cleanses may not be safe for individuals with cancer. It's essential to maintain adequate calorie and nutrient intake.

Monitor Side Effects: Some cancer treatments can cause digestive issues. Monitor how your body responds to juicing, and adjust your choices accordingly.

Hydration: Stay well-hydrated with water in addition to your juices.

Remember that juicing should complement your overall diet and not replace whole foods. Nutrient-rich whole foods provide a wide range of health benefits and fiber, which is essential for digestion. It's crucial to work closely with a healthcare professional to develop a dietary plan that suits your specific needs and the stage of cancer you're dealing with.

Chapter3:
Cancer-Fighting

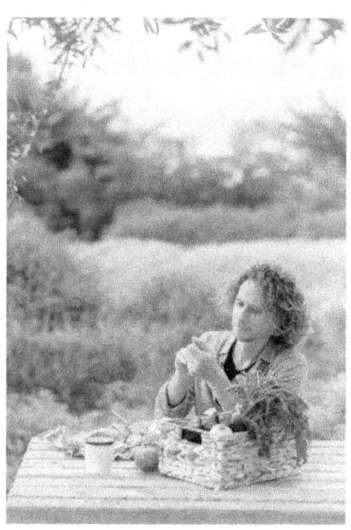

Ingredients

There are several ingredients that are known for their potential cancer-fighting properties. Some of them include:

Turmeric: Contains curcumin, a compound with anti-inflammatory and antioxidant effects.

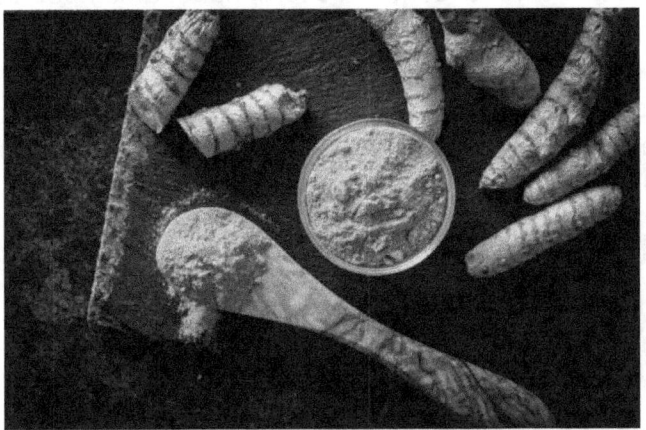

Green Tea: Rich in polyphenols like catechins, which have been studied for their cancer-preventive properties.

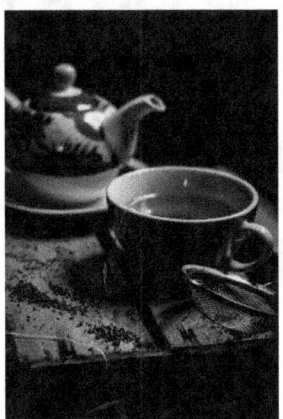

Cruciferous Vegetables: Broccoli, cauliflower, kale, and Brussels sprouts contain sulforaphane, a compound that may help protect against certain types of cancer.

Berries: Blueberries, strawberries, and raspberries are high in antioxidants, which can help combat oxidative stress linked to cancer.

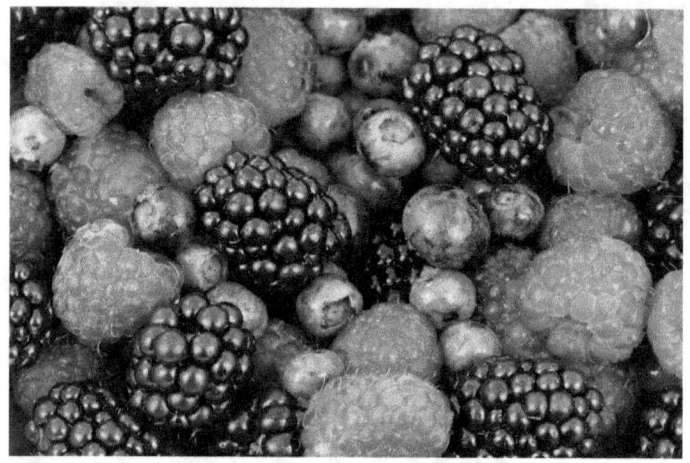

Garlic: Contains sulfur compounds that may have anti-cancer effects.

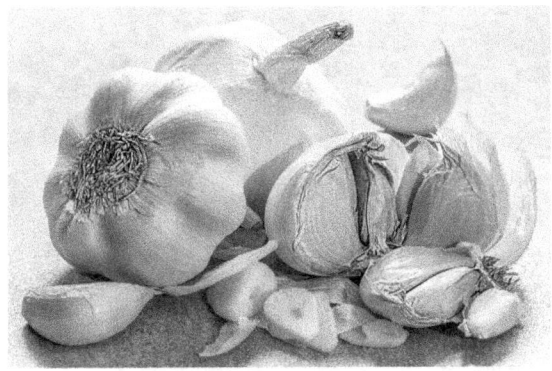

Ginger: Contains gingerol, which has anti-inflammatory and antioxidant properties.

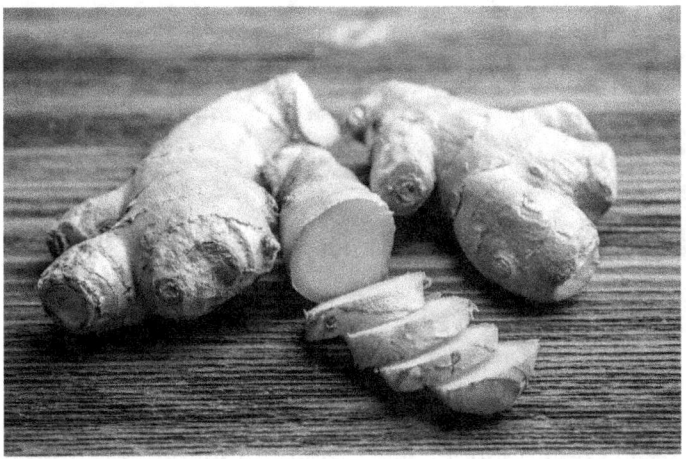

Tomatoes: Rich in lycopene, a powerful antioxidant that may reduce the risk of certain cancers.

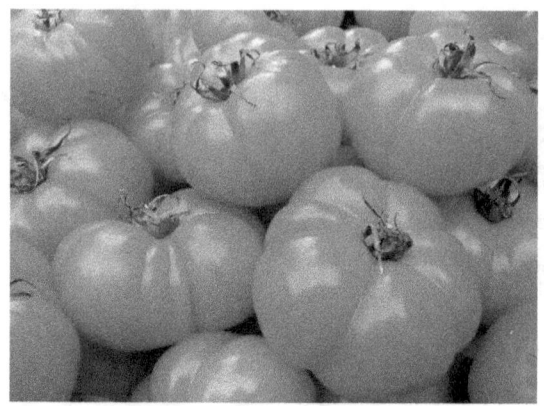

Fish with Omega-3 Fatty Acids: Such as salmon, mackerel, and sardines, which have anti-inflammatory properties.

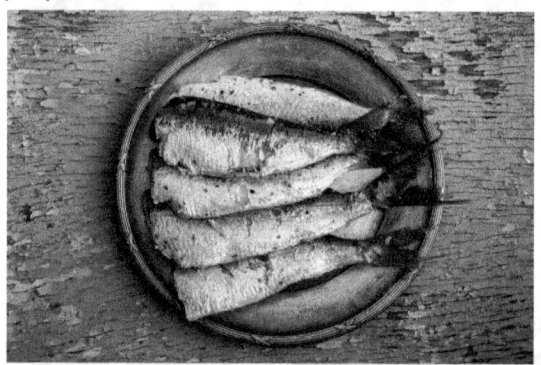

Mushrooms: Some types, like shiitake and maitake, contain compounds that may enhance the immune system and have anti-cancer potential.

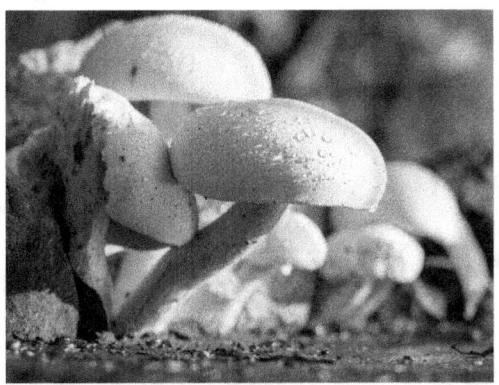

Fruits and Vegetables: In general, a diet rich in a variety of colorful fruits and vegetables provides a range of antioxidants and nutrients that can support overall health and potentially reduce cancer risk.

It's important to note that while these ingredients may have cancer-fighting properties, they should be part of a balanced and healthy diet. Consult with a healthcare professional for personalized advice regarding cancer prevention and treatment

Antioxidants and Their Role in Cancer Prevention

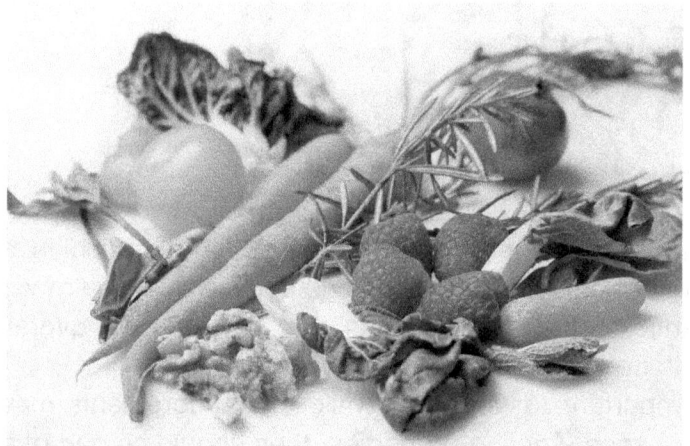

While advances in medical research have led to improved treatments, prevention remains a critical focus. Antioxidants have garnered considerable attention in the realm of cancer prevention due to their potential to combat oxidative stress, a process implicated in the development and progression of cancer. In this comprehensive content, we delve into the world of antioxidants and their pivotal role in cancer prevention.

Understanding Oxidative Stress

To appreciate the significance of antioxidants, one must first understand oxidative stress. It occurs when there is an imbalance between reactive oxygen species (ROS), commonly known as free radicals, and the body's antioxidant defenses. ROS are highly reactive molecules that, when present in excess, can damage cellular components such as DNA, proteins, and lipids. This oxidative damage can trigger mutations and contribute to the initiation of cancer.

The Role of Antioxidants

Antioxidants are molecules that counteract oxidative stress by neutralizing ROS. They work by donating electrons to free radicals, thus preventing them from causing cellular damage. The body produces its own antioxidants, including enzymes like superoxide dismutase and catalase, as well as non-enzymatic antioxidants such as glutathione. Additionally, antioxidants can be obtained from dietary sources, including vitamins (e.g., vitamin C and vitamin E), minerals (e.g., selenium), and various phytochemicals found in fruits and vegetables.

Antioxidants in Cancer Prevention

Antioxidants play a multifaceted role in cancer prevention:

DNA Protection: By preventing oxidative damage to DNA, antioxidants reduce the likelihood of mutations that could lead to cancerous transformations.

Inhibition of Tumor Growth: Some antioxidants have been found to inhibit the growth of tumor cells and promote their apoptosis (programmed cell death), which is crucial in preventing cancer progression.

Immune System Support: Antioxidants support the immune system's ability to recognize and eliminate cancer cells, bolstering the body's natural defenses.

Anti-Inflammatory Effects: Chronic inflammation is closely linked to cancer development. Antioxidants can mitigate inflammation, reducing the risk of cancer.

Detoxification: Antioxidants like glutathione aid in detoxifying harmful substances, potentially limiting their cancer-promoting effects.

Balanced Antioxidant Intake

While antioxidants hold promise in cancer prevention, balance is key. Excessive antioxidant supplementation may not always yield benefits and, in some cases, might even be harmful. For example, high-dose antioxidant supplements may interfere with chemotherapy or radiation therapy's effectiveness.

The best approach to harness the cancer-preventive potential of antioxidants is to maintain a diverse and balanced diet rich in fruits, vegetables, nuts, and seeds, which naturally provide antioxidants in appropriate quantities. This dietary strategy not only supplies antioxidants but also offers a wide array of other beneficial nutrients and compounds that can contribute to overall health.

Phytonutrients and Their Healing Properties

Phytonutrients, also known as phytochemicals, are natural compounds found in plants that offer a wide range of health benefits. These bioactive substances not only provide vibrant colors and distinctive flavors to fruits, vegetables, and other plant-based foods but also play a crucial role in promoting human health. In this comprehensive content, we'll delve into the fascinating world of phytonutrients and explore their diverse healing properties.

What are Phytonutrients?

Phytonutrients are non-nutritive compounds found in plants. Unlike macronutrients (carbohydrates, proteins, and fats) and micronutrients (vitamins and minerals), phytonutrients are not essential for basic human survival. However, they are increasingly recognized for their significant impact on overall health and well-being.

Types of Phytonutrients

There are thousands of different phytonutrients, each with its own unique properties and potential health benefits. Some of the most well-known phytonutrient groups include:

Flavonoids: These are antioxidants found in a variety of foods such as berries, citrus fruits, onions, and tea. Flavonoids have anti-inflammatory, antioxidant, and immune-boosting properties.

Carotenoids: Carotenoids give fruits and vegetables their vibrant colors. Beta-carotene, lutein, and zeaxanthin are notable examples. They support eye health and may reduce the risk of certain chronic diseases.

Glucosinolates: Found in cruciferous vegetables like broccoli, cauliflower, and kale, glucosinolates may have cancer-fighting properties.

Polyphenols: This diverse group includes resveratrol (found in red wine), quercetin (in apples and onions), and curcumin (in turmeric). Polyphenols have potent antioxidant and anti-inflammatory effects.

Lignans: These are found in seeds like flaxseeds and sesame seeds and may have cardiovascular benefits.

Healing Properties of Phytonutrients

Antioxidant Protection: Many phytonutrients, particularly flavonoids and polyphenols, act as antioxidants, helping to neutralize harmful free radicals in the body. This can reduce oxidative stress and lower the risk of chronic diseases like heart disease, cancer, and diabetes.

Anti-Inflammatory Effects: Certain phytonutrients, such as curcumin in turmeric, possess powerful anti-inflammatory properties. They may help alleviate symptoms of inflammatory conditions like arthritis.

Cancer Prevention: Phytonutrients like sulforaphane in broccoli and lycopene in tomatoes have been associated with a reduced risk of cancer.

Heart Health: Many phytonutrients, including resveratrol in red wine and flavonoids in dark chocolate, promote cardiovascular health by reducing cholesterol levels and improving blood vessel function.

Eye Protection: Carotenoids like lutein and zeaxanthin protect the eyes from age-related macular degeneration and cataracts.

Digestive Health: Fiber-rich foods containing phytonutrients can promote healthy digestion and reduce the risk of digestive disorders.

Brain Health: Some phytonutrients, like anthocyanins in berries, may support cognitive function and reduce the risk of age-related cognitive decline.

Immune-Boosting Ingredients

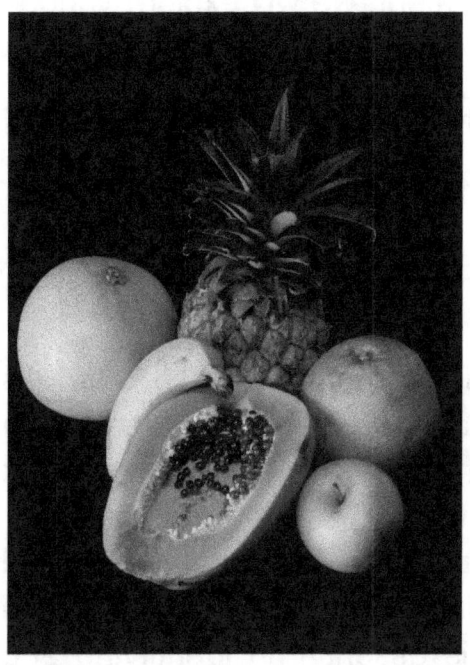

Cancer remains one of the most formidable health challenges of our time, with millions of lives affected worldwide. While advancements in cancer treatment have come a long way, prevention and immune support are vital aspects of the battle against this disease. Immune-boosting ingredients have gained significant attention for their potential role in reducing cancer risk and supporting cancer patients. In this comprehensive content, we will explore various immune-boosting ingredients and their relationship with cancer prevention and management.

Section 1: The Immune System and Cancer

Before delving into specific ingredients, it's crucial to understand the immune system's role in cancer. Our immune system is a complex network of cells, tissues, and organs that work together to defend the body against harmful invaders, including cancer cells. A strong immune system is essential in identifying and eliminating cancerous cells.

Section 2: Immune-Boosting Ingredients

Vitamin D:Vitamin D plays a pivotal role in immune function and may reduce the risk of certain cancers.
It supports the immune system by regulating immune cell activity and reducing inflammation.

Antioxidants:Antioxidants like vitamin C, vitamin E, and selenium help protect cells from damage caused by free radicals, potentially preventing cell mutations that can lead to cancer.

These antioxidants can be found in fruits, vegetables, and nuts.

Medicinal Mushrooms:Mushrooms like reishi, maitake, and shiitake contain beta-glucans and other compounds that enhance immune function.

They may help cancer patients by improving immune response and reducing side effects of treatments.

Green Tea:Green tea contains polyphenols, such as epigallocatechin gallate (EGCG), which have anti-inflammatory and antioxidant properties.

Studies suggest that green tea consumption may reduce the risk of certain cancers.

Turmeric and Curcumin:Curcumin, the active compound in turmeric, has anti-inflammatory and antioxidant properties.

It may help inhibit the growth of cancer cells and reduce inflammation in the body.

Section 3: Cancer Prevention and Support

Dietary Choices:A balanced diet rich in immune-boosting ingredients can support overall health and reduce cancer risk.
Emphasizing fruits, vegetables, whole grains, and lean proteins is essential.

Lifestyle Factors:Regular exercise, stress management, and adequate sleep play crucial roles in maintaining a healthy immune system and reducing cancer risk.

Integrative Approaches:

Integrative medicine combines conventional treatments with complementary therapies like acupuncture, massage, and dietary supplements to support cancer patients.

Alkaline Foods and Their Importance

Cancer is a relentless adversary that affects millions of lives worldwide. While medical treatments are pivotal in the battle against cancer, the importance of diet in supporting cancer patients cannot be understated. In recent years, the concept of alkaline foods and their potential benefits for cancer patients has garnered significant attention. This comprehensive content aims to explore the significance of alkaline foods in the context of cancer, shedding light on their potential to aid in the fight against this devastating disease.

Understanding Alkaline Foods:

Alkaline foods, often referred to as alkaline-forming foods, are those that have an alkalizing effect on the body when metabolized. They typically have a pH value above 7.0 and are rich in minerals like potassium, magnesium, and calcium. These foods play a crucial role in maintaining the body's pH balance, which is essential for overall health.

The Alkaline Diet and Cancer:

Research suggests that the pH level of the body can influence cancer development and progression. While cancer cells thrive in an acidic environment, an alkaline environment may inhibit their growth. This forms the basis of the alkaline diet's connection to cancer.

Importance of Alkaline Foods for Cancer Patients:

Balancing pH Levels: Alkaline foods help maintain a slightly alkaline pH in the body, creating an environment less conducive to cancer cell proliferation.

Reducing Inflammation:

Many alkaline foods are anti-inflammatory, which can be beneficial for cancer patients as chronic inflammation is often linked to cancer.

Enhancing Immunity:

Alkaline foods are often rich in essential vitamins, minerals, and antioxidants that boost the immune system. A robust immune system is vital for cancer patients undergoing treatment.

Supporting Detoxification:

Some alkaline foods, like leafy greens, aid in the body's natural detoxification processes, helping eliminate harmful toxins that could contribute to cancer.

Weight Management:

Maintaining a healthy weight is crucial for cancer patients, and alkaline foods can support weight management due to their low-calorie and nutrient-dense nature.

Alkaline Foods to Include:

Leafy greens (spinach, kale)

Cruciferous vegetables (broccoli, cauliflower)

Chapter4: Juicing Recipes for Specific Types of Cancer

medical treatments play a crucial role in cancer management, nutrition also plays a significant part in supporting the body during this battle. Juicing, a method of extracting and consuming the concentrated nutrients from fruits and vegetables, can be a valuable addition to a cancer patient's diet. In this comprehensive guide, we'll explore juicing recipes tailored to specific types of cancer, aiming to provide essential nutrients and promote overall well-being.

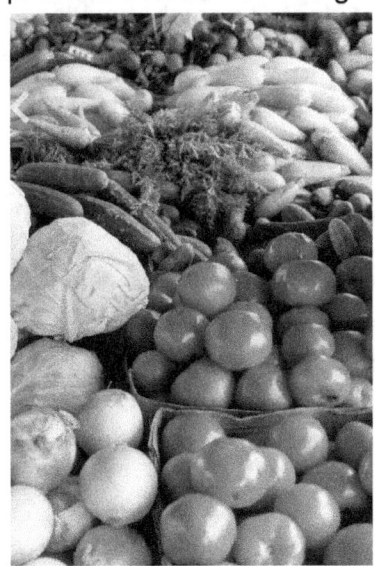

Breast Cancer:
Breast cancer is one of the most common forms of cancer among women. To support breast cancer patients, these juicing recipes can provide antioxidants, vitamins, and phytonutrients known to benefit breast health:

a. Green Goddess Juice:
- Ingredients: Spinach, kale, cucumber, green apples, and ginger.
- Benefits: Rich in chlorophyll, vitamin C, and folate to support the immune system and reduce inflammation.

b. **Berry Bliss Juice:**
- Ingredients: Blueberries, raspberries, strawberries, and a hint of lemon.
- Benefits: Packed with antioxidants to combat oxidative stress and support overall health.

Prostate Cancer:
Prostate cancer predominantly affects men.
Incorporating these juicing recipes into the diet can help provide nutrients beneficial for prostate health:

a. Prostate Protector Juice:
- Ingredients: Tomatoes, carrots, watermelon, and a touch of basil.
- Benefits: Contains lycopene, a powerful antioxidant associated with prostate health.

b. Green Tea Infused Juice:
- Ingredients: Green tea, cucumber, and mint leaves.
- Benefits: Green tea is rich in catechins that may help reduce the risk of prostate cancer.

Colon Cancer:
Colon cancer is often linked to dietary factors. These juicing recipes can promote colon health and provide essential nutrients:

a. Colon Cleansing Juice:
- Ingredients: Spinach, celery, ginger, and aloe vera gel.
- Benefits: Supports digestion, reduces inflammation, and provides essential vitamins.

b. Fiber-Packed Delight:
- Ingredients: Apples, pears, broccoli, and chia seeds.
- Benefits: High in fiber to promote healthy bowel movements and reduce the risk of colon cancer.

Lung Cancer:
Lung cancer is commonly associated with smoking, but nutrition can still play a role. These juicing recipes focus on lung health:

a. Carrot and Ginger Elixir:
- Ingredients: Carrots, ginger, and a hint of turmeric.
- **Benefits**: Rich in beta-carotene and anti-inflammatory compounds to support lung function.

b. Citrus Boost Juice:

- Ingredients: Oranges, grapefruits, and a touch of mint.
- **Benefits**: Provides vitamin C and antioxidants to protect lung tissues.

Juicing for Breast Cancer

Breast cancer is a prevalent and life-altering disease affecting millions of women worldwide. While medical treatments play a crucial role in managing breast cancer, adopting a healthy lifestyle and diet can complement traditional therapies. Juicing, a practice of extracting fresh fruit and vegetable juices, has gained attention for its potential health benefits, including its role in supporting breast cancer patients. In this comprehensive guide, we will explore the relationship between juicing and breast cancer, highlighting the potential advantages, considerations, and recipes to aid those on their breast cancer journey.

The Benefits of Juicing for Breast Cancer:

Nutrient-Rich Support: Freshly squeezed juices are a concentrated source of essential vitamins, minerals, and antioxidants. These nutrients can support overall health and help bolster the immune system, which is vital for cancer patients.

Hydration: Staying hydrated is crucial during cancer treatment. Juices can provide a delicious and easy way to increase fluid intake, helping combat the dehydration often associated with chemotherapy and radiation therapy.

Digestive Ease: Some breast cancer treatments can lead to digestive issues such as nausea or difficulty in swallowing. Juices can be a gentle way to nourish the body without putting extra stress on the digestive system.

Weight Management: Maintaining a healthy weight is important during and after breast cancer treatment. Juicing can provide a low-calorie option for those looking to manage their weight.

Considerations When Juicing for Breast Cancer:

Consult Your Healthcare Team: Always consult with your oncologist or healthcare provider before making significant dietary changes.

Choose the Right Ingredients: Opt for fruits and vegetables rich in cancer-fighting compounds like antioxidants and phytochemicals. Examples include broccoli, kale, carrots, berries, and citrus fruits.

Be Mindful of Sugar Content: While natural sugars in fruits are generally healthy, excessive sugar intake can be detrimental. Balance fruit and vegetable choices to avoid excessive sugar consumption.

Ensure Food Safety: Wash fruits and vegetables thoroughly to reduce the risk of foodborne illnesses. Consider using organic produce whenever possible.

Juicing Recipes for Breast Cancer Support:

Green Powerhouse Juice:

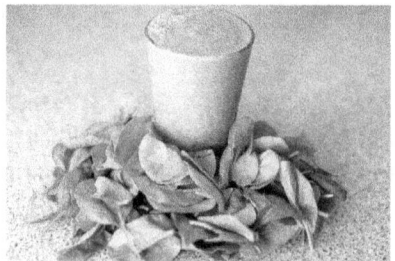

Ingredients: Kale, spinach, cucumber, green apple, lemon, ginger.
Benefits: Packed with antioxidants, this juice provides a nutrient boost and supports overall well-being.

Berry Bliss Juice:

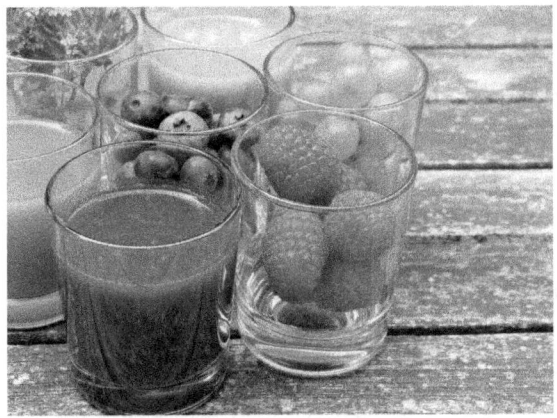

Ingredients: Blueberries, strawberries, raspberries, kale, spinach, lemon.
Benefits: Rich in anti-inflammatory compounds and vitamin C, this juice can help boost immunity.
Carrot & Turmeric Elixir:

Ingredients: Carrots, turmeric root, oranges, ginger.
Benefits: Turmeric's anti-inflammatory properties combined with vitamin C from oranges make this juice a powerful choice.

Juicing for Lung Cancer

Lung cancer is a devastating disease that affects millions of people worldwide. While medical treatments are essential, adopting a healthy diet can play a supportive role in managing the condition. Juicing, which involves extracting the liquid from fruits and vegetables, is a popular dietary approach that may offer benefits for individuals with lung cancer. In this comprehensive guide, we'll explore the potential benefits of juicing, provide recipes, and offer tips for incorporating juicing into a lung cancer management plan.

Benefits of Juicing for Lung Cancer Patients

Nutrient Density: Freshly made juices are packed with essential nutrients like vitamins, minerals, and antioxidants. These nutrients are crucial for overall health and can help strengthen the immune system, which is particularly important for lung cancer patients.

Hydration: Proper hydration is essential during cancer treatment. Juices provide hydration while delivering nutrients that can be lost during therapy, such as chemotherapy.

Digestive Ease: Juices are easier to digest than whole fruits and vegetables. They can be beneficial for individuals with reduced appetite or digestive issues often associated with cancer treatments.

Antioxidant Support: Many fruits and vegetables used in juicing contain antioxidants like vitamin C, which can help combat oxidative stress and reduce inflammation in the body.

Juicing Tips for Lung Cancer Patients

Consult a Healthcare Professional: Always consult with your oncologist or a registered dietitian before making significant dietary changes, including juicing, to ensure it's safe and suitable for your specific condition and treatment plan.

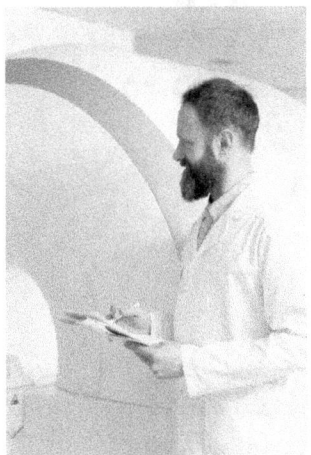

Choose Organic: Whenever possible, select organic produce to reduce exposure to pesticides and chemicals.

Variety is Key: Incorporate a variety of fruits and vegetables into your juices to ensure a broad spectrum of nutrients. Different colors represent different types of antioxidants and phytochemicals.

Moderation: While juicing can be beneficial, it's important not to rely solely on juices for nutrition. A balanced diet that includes whole foods is crucial.

Monitor Sugar Intake: Some fruits can be high in natural sugars. Be mindful of your sugar intake, especially if you have concerns about blood sugar levels.

Juice Recipes for Lung Cancer Patients

Green Detox Juice:

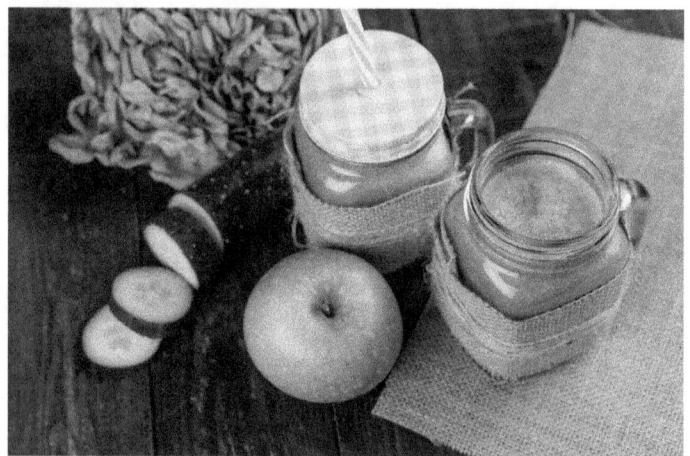

Ingredients: Spinach, kale, cucumber, celery, lemon, and ginger.
Benefits: Rich in chlorophyll, vitamins, and antioxidants for detoxification and immune support.
Carrot-Orange Immunity Booster:

Ingredients: Carrots, oranges, turmeric, and a touch of black pepper.
Benefits: High in vitamin C and anti-inflammatory properties to support the immune system.
Berry Blast:

Ingredients: Blueberries, strawberries, raspberries, and a bit of spinach.

Benefits: Packed with antioxidants and vitamins for overall health.

Beetroot Cleanse:

Ingredients: Beets, apples, carrots, and a hint of lemon.

Benefits: Supports detoxification and provides essential nutrients.

Conclusion

While juicing can be a valuable addition to the diet of lung cancer patients, it should not replace conventional medical treatments or a balanced diet. It's essential to work closely with healthcare professionals to ensure that juicing is safe and appropriate for your individual circumstances. A combination of medical care, a well-balanced diet, and healthy lifestyle choices can help support lung cancer patients on their journey toward better health and well-being.

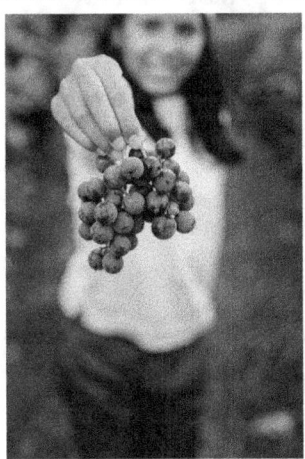

Juicing for Prostate Cancer

Prostate cancer is a prevalent health concern among men worldwide, with early detection and prevention playing a crucial role in managing this condition. While there is no surefire way to prevent prostate cancer, adopting a healthy lifestyle that includes a balanced diet can significantly reduce the risk. Juicing, in particular, has gained popularity as a natural approach to support prostate health. In this comprehensive guide, we'll explore the benefits of juicing for prostate cancer, recommended ingredients, and some delicious recipes to get you started.

The Role of Nutrition:
Nutrition plays a pivotal role in the development and progression of prostate cancer. Certain dietary factors have been linked to an increased risk, such as a high intake of saturated fats and red meat. On the other hand, consuming fruits and vegetables rich in antioxidants, vitamins, and minerals can help reduce the risk of prostate cancer and support overall prostate health.

Benefits of Juicing:
Juicing is an efficient way to pack a variety of nutrients into one glass. Here are some specific benefits of juicing for prostate cancer:

Antioxidant Power: Fruits and vegetables like berries, spinach, kale, and carrots are rich in antioxidants that combat oxidative stress, a key factor in cancer development.

Anti-Inflammatory Properties: Ginger and turmeric are potent anti-inflammatory ingredients that can help reduce inflammation in the prostate.

Immune System Support: Vitamin C from citrus fruits and zinc from pumpkin seeds are essential for a robust immune system, which can aid in cancer prevention and recovery.

Hydration: Proper hydration is essential for overall health, and fresh juices contribute to your daily fluid intake.

Recommended Ingredients:

When juicing for prostate health, consider including these ingredients:

Berries (blueberries, strawberries, raspberries)

Leafy greens (kale, spinach)

Cruciferous vegetables (broccoli, cauliflower)

Tomatoes

Carrots

Celery

Ginger

Turmeric

Citrus fruits (oranges, lemons)

Pumpkin seeds (for zinc)

Delicious Juicing Recipes:

Here are two prostate-friendly juice recipes to get you started:

Prostate Protector Juice:

1 cup of kale
1/2 cup of blueberries
1 medium tomato
1/2 inch piece of ginger
1 tablespoon of pumpkin seeds
Juice all ingredients and enjoy!
Citrus Delight:

2 oranges
1 lemon
1/2 inch piece of turmeric
1 carrot
Juice the fruits and carrot, then add freshly grated
turmeric. Mix and serve.

Juicing for Colon Cancer

Colon cancer is a serious health concern affecting
millions of people worldwide. While traditional medical
treatments play a crucial role in managing this disease,
incorporating a well-balanced diet can complement your
treatment plan. Juicing, the process of extracting fresh
juices from fruits and vegetables, offers a convenient
and delicious way to boost your nutritional intake. In this
comprehensive guide, we'll explore the potential benefits
of juicing for colon cancer patients, the best ingredients

to include, and some essential tips for safe and effective juicing.

The Benefits of Juicing for Colon Cancer

Nutrient-Rich Diet: Colon cancer treatment can deplete your body of essential nutrients. Freshly juiced fruits and vegetables are packed with vitamins, minerals, and antioxidants that can help support your overall health.

Hydration: Maintaining proper hydration is vital during cancer treatment. Juices are an excellent source of hydration, especially for those who may have difficulty drinking large amounts of water.

Digestive Support: Certain fruits and vegetables, like ginger and aloe vera, can soothe the digestive tract and ease discomfort often associated with colon cancer and its treatments.

Increased Energy: Juicing can provide a quick and easily digestible source of energy, helping you combat fatigue, a common side effect of cancer therapy.

Best Ingredients for Juicing

Dark Leafy Greens: Kale, spinach, and Swiss chard are rich in folate and fiber, which may help support colon health.

Cruciferous Vegetables: Broccoli, cauliflower, and Brussels sprouts contain compounds that have been linked to cancer prevention.

Colorful Fruits: Berries, citrus fruits, and papaya are loaded with antioxidants like vitamin C, which
can help protect cells from damage.

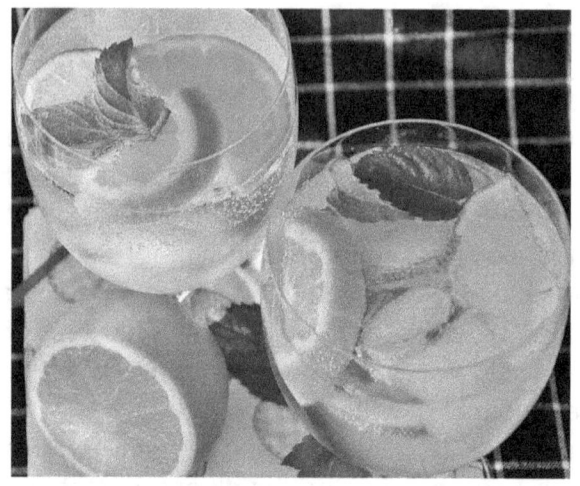

Ginger and Turmeric: These anti-inflammatory spices can provide relief from digestive discomfort and may have potential anti-cancer properties.

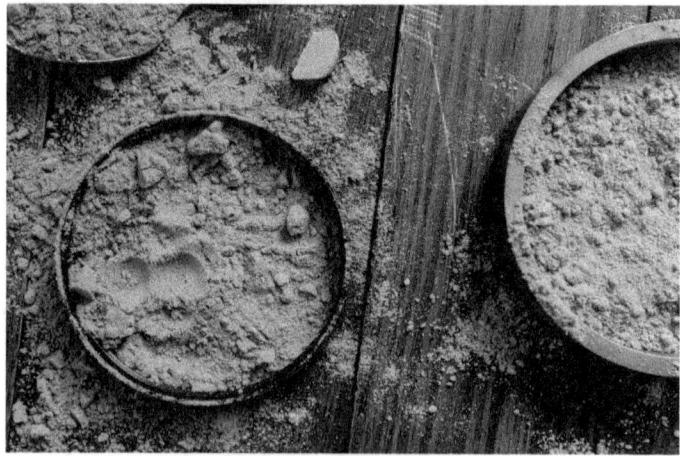

Aloe Vera: Known for its soothing properties, aloe vera can be added to your juice to help ease digestive issues.

Carrots: Carrots are an excellent source of beta-carotene, which can promote immune health.

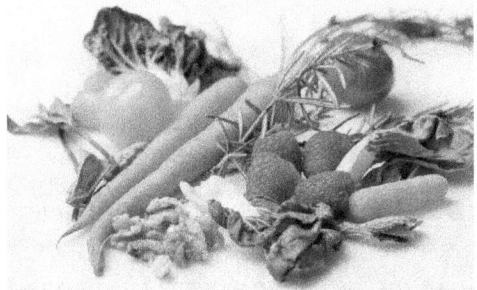

Apples: Apples add natural sweetness to your juices and provide dietary fiber.

Juicing Tips for Colon Cancer Patients
Consult Your Healthcare Provider: Always discuss dietary changes, including juicing, with your healthcare team to ensure it aligns with your treatment plan.

Use Organic Produce: Whenever possible, choose organic fruits and vegetables to minimize exposure to pesticides and chemicals.

Variety is Key: Rotate your ingredients to benefit from a wide range of nutrients. Avoid excessive consumption of any one ingredient.

Maintain Proper Hygiene: Thoroughly wash all produce before juicing to reduce the risk of contamination.

Monitor Sugar Intake: Be mindful of the sugar content in your juices, especially if you have diabetes or are concerned about blood sugar levels.

Start Slowly: If you're new to juicing, start with small servings and gradually increase them to assess how your body responds.

Juicing for Ovarian Cancer

Ovarian cancer is a formidable adversary, affecting thousands of women each year. While medical treatments are vital in the fight against this disease, complementary approaches to enhance well-being and support the body's natural defenses have gained increasing attention. Juicing, a practice that involves extracting the liquid content from fruits and vegetables, is one such approach that offers potential benefits for individuals dealing with ovarian cancer. In this comprehensive guide, we will explore the role of juicing in managing ovarian cancer, the best ingredients to include in your juices, and the precautions to take.

Understanding Ovarian Cancer

Ovarian cancer is known for its stealthy nature, often presenting with subtle or vague symptoms in its early stages. This makes early detection challenging, and many cases are diagnosed at advanced stages. Treatment typically involves surgery, chemotherapy, and sometimes radiation therapy. However, patients often face side effects and challenges related to these treatments, making the need for complementary therapies evident.

The Potential Benefits of Juicing

Juicing, when done right, can be a valuable addition to an ovarian cancer patient's journey. **Here are some potential benefits:**

Nutrient Boost: Freshly prepared juices can provide a concentrated source of essential nutrients, including vitamins, minerals, antioxidants, and phytochemicals. These nutrients support overall health and can help combat treatment-related side effects.

Hydration: Maintaining proper hydration is crucial during cancer treatment. Juices can contribute to your daily fluid intake, keeping you hydrated and supporting bodily functions.

Digestive Ease: For some cancer patients, treatment can lead to digestive issues. Juices, particularly those made from easily digestible fruits and vegetables, can be gentler on the stomach.

Weight Management: Ovarian cancer and its treatments can affect appetite and weight. Nutrient-dense juices can help manage weight and provide energy.

Choosing the Right Ingredients

When juicing for ovarian cancer, selecting the right ingredients is paramount. Here are some recommendations:

Dark Leafy Greens: Kale, spinach, and Swiss chard are rich in antioxidants and can boost immunity.

Colorful Vegetables: Carrots, beets, and bell peppers provide a spectrum of vitamins and minerals.

Anti-Inflammatory Fruits: Berries, citrus fruits, and pineapple contain anti-inflammatory compounds.

Turmeric and Ginger: These spices have anti-inflammatory properties and may help manage nausea.

Hydration with Cucumber: Cucumber-based juices can aid in hydration.

Protein Sources: Add some nuts, seeds, or yogurt to increase protein content.

Precautions and Considerations

While juicing offers many benefits, it's essential to exercise caution:

Consult Your Healthcare Team: Always discuss juicing with your healthcare provider to ensure it complements your treatment plan.

Food Safety: Ensure the cleanliness of ingredients and equipment to minimize the risk of foodborne illnesses.

Sugar Content: Limit fruits high in sugar to avoid blood sugar spikes.

Variety is Key: Rotate ingredients to ensure a diverse intake of nutrients.

Moderation: Do not rely solely on juices; they should be part of a balanced diet.

Juicing for Blood Cancers (Leukemia, Lymphoma)

Blood cancers, such as leukemia and lymphoma, can be physically and emotionally challenging for patients. While medical treatments like chemotherapy, radiation, and stem cell transplants are essential components of the treatment plan, adopting a healthy lifestyle and nutrition strategy can play a complementary role in managing the disease. Juicing, a popular trend in the wellness world, has gained attention for its potential benefits in aiding cancer patients. In this comprehensive content, we will explore the potential advantages of juicing for individuals battling leukemia and lymphoma, keeping in mind that it should always be part of an overall treatment plan under the guidance of healthcare professionals.

Understanding Leukemia and Lymphoma:

Leukemia and lymphoma are types of blood cancers that affect the body's lymphatic system and bone marrow. They disrupt the production of healthy blood cells, leading to various symptoms, including fatigue, anemia, bruising, and susceptibility to infections. The treatment for these cancers often involves chemotherapy, radiation, and, in some cases, stem cell transplantation.

The Role of Nutrition:

Nutrition is a critical aspect of cancer care. Maintaining a well-balanced diet can help boost the immune system, manage side effects of treatment, and enhance overall well-being. Juicing, the process of extracting liquid from fruits and vegetables, is a convenient way to provide the body with essential nutrients.

Benefits of Juicing for Blood Cancer Patients:

Nutrient Density: Juicing allows patients to consume a concentrated source of vitamins, minerals, and antioxidants found in fruits and vegetables. These nutrients can support the immune system, which is often compromised during cancer treatment.

Hydration: Staying well-hydrated is essential for cancer patients. Juices provide a source of hydration while also supplying nutrients that water alone cannot provide.

Digestive Relief: Some cancer treatments may cause digestive discomfort. Juices can be easier to digest and can provide relief from nausea or mouth sores, common side effects of chemotherapy.

Energy Boost: The vitamins and minerals in fresh juices can help combat cancer-related fatigue, enabling patients to maintain a higher level of energy throughout treatment.

Weight Management: Maintaining a healthy weight is crucial for cancer patients. Juicing can be a way to get essential nutrients without overloading the digestive system, making it suitable for patients who may have difficulty eating solid foods.

Choosing the Right Ingredients:

When juicing for blood cancer patients, it's important to select ingredients that align with their specific nutritional needs:

Dark leafy greens: Kale, spinach, and Swiss chard are rich in vitamins, minerals, and antioxidants.

Cruciferous vegetables: Broccoli, cauliflower, and Brussels sprouts may have cancer-fighting properties.

Berries: Blueberries, strawberries, and raspberries provide antioxidants and vitamins.

Citrus fruits: Oranges, grapefruits, and lemons offer vitamin C and immune support.

Carrots: High in beta-carotene, which the body converts to vitamin A.

Ginger and turmeric: Known for their anti-inflammatory properties.

Precautions and Consultation:

While juicing can offer numerous benefits, it's essential for blood cancer patients to approach it with caution:

Avoid excessive sugar: Be mindful of the sugar content in juices, as excessive sugar intake can be detrimental to cancer patients. Focus on vegetables and low-sugar fruits.

Food safety: Ensure that all ingredients are thoroughly washed and that the juicing equipment is clean to prevent infection.

Individualized approach: The nutritional needs of cancer patients can vary widely. Customize juice recipes based on the patient's specific condition, treatment, and dietary restrictions.

Juicing for Skin Cancer

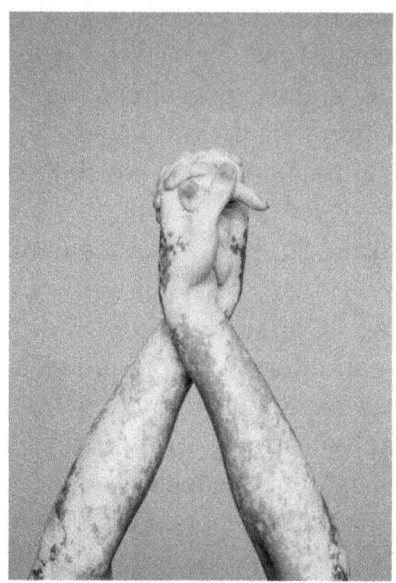

Skin cancer is a prevalent and concerning health issue, affecting millions of people worldwide. While medical treatments and therapies are essential in managing skin cancer, incorporating a holistic approach to wellness can play a supportive role in the overall treatment process. Juicing, with its abundance of nutrients and antioxidants, has gained attention as a potential adjunctive therapy for individuals dealing with skin cancer. In this comprehensive content, we will explore the benefits of juicing for skin cancer, its potential impact on prevention, and important considerations when incorporating juicing into your routine.

Understanding Skin Cancer:

Skin cancer is a condition characterized by the abnormal growth of skin cells. It can manifest in various forms, including basal cell carcinoma, squamous cell carcinoma, and melanoma. The primary risk factors for skin cancer include exposure to ultraviolet (UV) radiation, genetics, and a compromised immune system. Prevention, early detection, and comprehensive medical treatment are crucial aspects of managing this disease.

The Role of Nutrition in Skin Health:

Proper nutrition is essential for maintaining skin health and supporting the body's ability to combat diseases like skin cancer. Nutrients such as vitamins A, C, D, and E, as well as antioxidants like beta-carotene and lycopene, play vital roles in skin maintenance, repair, and protection against UV radiation. These nutrients are abundant in fruits and vegetables, making juicing an attractive option for those seeking to enhance their nutritional intake.

Benefits of Juicing for Skin Cancer:

Nutrient Density: Juicing provides a concentrated source of essential nutrients, ensuring that your body receives a high dose of vitamins, minerals, and antioxidants that are beneficial for skin health.

Hydration: Proper hydration is critical for skin health. Juices, made primarily from water-rich fruits and vegetables, help keep your skin well-hydrated, promoting elasticity and overall health.

Antioxidants: Antioxidants found in fruits and vegetables can help combat free radicals, which are implicated in the development of skin cancer. They protect skin cells from oxidative damage.

Immune Support: A strong immune system is essential in fighting cancer. Nutrient-rich juices can bolster your immune response, aiding the body in recognizing and eliminating cancerous cells.

Inflammation Reduction: Chronic inflammation is associated with the progression of cancer. Juices with anti-inflammatory properties can help reduce inflammation and promote healing.

Selecting the Right Ingredients:

When juicing for skin cancer, it's essential to choose ingredients that are not only delicious but also packed with skin-loving nutrients. Some excellent choices include:

Leafy greens like kale and spinach for vitamin A and C.

Citrus fruits such as oranges and lemons for vitamin C.Carrots for beta-carotene.

Berries like blueberries and strawberries for antioxidants.

Cruciferous vegetables like broccoli and cauliflower for their cancer-fighting properties.

Caution and Considerations:

While juicing can be a valuable addition to a skin cancer management plan, it should not replace conventional medical treatments. Always consult with your healthcare provider before making significant dietary changes, especially if you are undergoing cancer treatment or taking medications.

Furthermore, it's essential to maintain a balanced diet that includes a variety of foods beyond juices to ensure you receive a wide range of nutrients necessary for your overall well-being.

Juicing for Brain Tumors

Brain tumor cancer is a devastating diagnosis that can significantly impact a person's life. While medical treatment is essential, proper nutrition plays a crucial role in supporting overall health and well-being during the journey to recovery. Juicing, with its concentrated nutrients, is an attractive option for individuals with brain tumors. This comprehensive guide explores the benefits of juicing for brain tumor cancer patients and provides valuable insights into incorporating juicing into a holistic approach to healing.

Understanding Brain Tumor Cancer

Brain tumor cancer is a complex condition that can affect different parts of the brain. It can lead to a variety of symptoms, including headaches, seizures, changes in personality, and cognitive difficulties. The treatment approach typically involves surgery, radiation therapy, chemotherapy, or a combination of these treatments, depending on the type and stage of the tumor.

The Role of Nutrition in Brain Tumor Cancer

Proper nutrition is vital for anyone battling cancer, as it helps maintain strength, supports the immune system, and aids in the recovery process. For brain tumor cancer patients, nutrition becomes even more critical due to potential side effects of treatment and the tumor's impact on cognitive function.

Benefits of Juicing

Juicing involves extracting the liquid and nutrients from fruits and vegetables, providing a concentrated source of vitamins, minerals, antioxidants, and phytochemicals. Here are some key benefits of incorporating juicing into the diet of brain tumor cancer patients:

Nutrient Density: Juicing allows patients to consume a high concentration of essential nutrients in an easily digestible form, which is particularly beneficial for those with reduced appetite or difficulty swallowing.

Hydration: Staying well-hydrated is crucial during cancer treatment. Fresh juices can help maintain proper hydration levels while providing essential nutrients.

Digestive Ease: The absence of fiber in juice makes it easier on the digestive system, reducing the risk of digestive discomfort or complications.

Antioxidant Support: Many fruits and vegetables used in juicing are rich in antioxidants, which help combat oxidative stress and inflammation, potentially reducing the risk of tumor progression.

Mental Clarity: Certain nutrients in fruits and vegetables, such as folate and vitamin K, are associated with improved cognitive function, which can be particularly important for brain tumor patients.

Juicing Recipes for Brain Tumor Cancer Patients

When juicing for brain tumor cancer patients, it's essential to prioritize nutrient-rich ingredients. Here are some suggested juice recipes:

Brain-Boosting Green Juice

Ingredients: Kale, spinach, cucumber, celery, apple, lemon

Benefits: Rich in antioxidants, vitamins, and minerals that support brain health.

Anti-Inflammatory Berry Blast

Ingredients: Blueberries, strawberries, ginger, turmeric, carrots, orange

Benefits: Reduces inflammation and provides immune-boosting antioxidants.

Immune Support Juice

Ingredients: Carrots, beets, ginger, garlic, lemon

Benefits: Supports the immune system and provides a nutritional boost.

Considerations and Precautions

While juicing can be highly beneficial, it's crucial to consult with a healthcare professional or registered dietitian before making significant dietary changes, especially during cancer treatment. Some **considerations include:**

Monitoring sugar intake to avoid excessive sugar content in juices.

Ensuring the safety of the ingredients, especially if the patient is immunocompromised.

Being mindful of potential interactions with medications.

Customizing juice recipes to meet the patient's specific nutritional needs.

Chapter5: Managing Side Effects

A cancer diagnosis can be a life-altering event, and the journey of battling cancer often comes with a range of challenging side effects caused by the disease itself or its treatments. Managing these side effects is crucial not only for the physical well-being of patients but also for their emotional and psychological health. In this guide, we will explore common side effects of cancer and offer practical strategies for effectively managing them.

Nausea and Vomiting:

Chemotherapy and radiation therapy can trigger nausea and vomiting. To manage these side effects, patients can:

Take anti-nausea medications as prescribed by their healthcare provider.

Opt for small, frequent meals.

Consume ginger or peppermint, known for their anti-nausea properties.

Stay well-hydrated.

Fatigue:

Cancer-related fatigue is a pervasive side effect.

Patients can combat fatigue by:

Prioritizing rest and sleep.

Engaging in light exercise, like walking or yoga.

Planning activities during periods of higher energy.

Seeking support from friends and family.

Hair Loss:

Hair loss is often associated with chemotherapy. Coping strategies include:

Considering wigs, scarves, or hats.

Embracing the beauty of a bald head.

Talking to a therapist or support group about body image concerns.

Pain:

Cancer-related pain can be managed with:

Pain medications prescribed by a healthcare provider.

Physical therapy or massage.

Relaxation techniques such as deep breathing and meditation.

Changes in Appetite and Taste:

Cancer and its treatments can alter taste and appetite. Patients can:

Experiment with different foods and flavors.

Maintain good oral hygiene.

Consult with a dietitian for personalized dietary recommendations.

Emotional and Psychological Distress:

Cancer can take a toll on mental health. Strategies to address this include:

Seeking support from therapists, counselors, or support groups.

Practicing mindfulness and relaxation techniques.

Sharing feelings and concerns with loved ones.

Neuropathy:

Chemotherapy-induced neuropathy can cause tingling and numbness. Patients can:

Report symptoms to their healthcare team.
Consider physical therapy or occupational therapy.
Use assistive devices if necessary.

Constipation and Diarrhea:

Digestive issues can arise during cancer treatment. To manage these, patients can:

Maintain hydration.

Follow dietary recommendations from healthcare providers.

Use over-the-counter remedies if advised.

Conclusion:

Managing the side effects of cancer requires a multidimensional approach that includes medical intervention, lifestyle adjustments, and emotional support. It's essential for patients to communicate openly with their healthcare team, follow prescribed treatments, and seek help when needed. With the right strategies and support, individuals can enhance their quality of life during their cancer journey. Remember that each person's experience is unique, so a personalized approach to managing side effects is key.

Nausea and Digestive Issues

Cancer is a complex and often devastating disease that can affect various parts of the body. Nausea and digestive issues are common side effects experienced by cancer patients, primarily due to the disease itself and the treatments used to combat it. These symptoms can significantly impact apatient's quality of life and overall well-being. In this comprehensive content, we will delve into the causes, symptoms, management, and coping strategies for nausea and digestive issues in relation to cancer.

Causes of Nausea and Digestive Issues in Cancer Patients:

A. Cancer Itself:

1. Tumors can interfere with the normal functioning of the digestive system.

2. Certain cancers, such as stomach or pancreatic cancer, may directly affect digestion.

B. **Cancer Treatments**:

1. **Chemotherapy**: Potent drugs used to kill cancer cells can irritate the stomach lining and trigger nausea.

2. **Radiation Therapy:** Radiation aimed at cancerous areas can harm nearby healthy tissues, including the digestive tract.

3. **Immunotherapy**: Some immune system-targeting therapies may lead to digestive side effects.

C. **Medications:**

1. Painkillers, antibiotics, or other medications commonly prescribed to cancer patients may cause nausea and digestive issues.

II. Symptoms of Nausea and Digestive Issues in Cancer Patients:

A. Nausea:

1. Persistent feeling of queasiness.

2. Vomiting.

3. Loss of appetite.

4. Weight loss.

B. Digestive Issues:
1. Diarrhea or constipation.
2. Abdominal pain or cramping.
3. Bloating and gas.
4. Acid reflux or heartburn.
III. Management of Nausea and Digestive Issues:
A. Medications:
1. Antiemetic drugs to control nausea and vomiting.
2. Proton pump inhibitors or antacids for acid reflux.
3. Laxatives or stool softeners for constipation.
B. Dietary Changes:
1. Eating smaller, more frequent meals.
2. Avoiding spicy, greasy, or heavy foods.
3. Opting for bland and easily digestible foods.
4. Staying hydrated.
C. Lifestyle Modifications:
1. Gentle exercise to promote digestion.
2. Stress-reduction techniques like meditation or yoga.
3. Adequate rest and sleep.
D. Alternative Therapies:
1. Acupuncture or acupressure for nausea relief.
2. Herbal teas, such as ginger or peppermint, known for their soothing effects on the digestive system.
IV. Coping Strategies for Cancer Patients:
A. Communication:
1. Open and honest discussions with healthcare providers about symptoms.
2. Seeking emotional support from friends, family, or support groups.
B. Preparing for Side Effects:

1. Being aware that nausea and digestive issues are common side effects can help patients mentally prepare for them.
2. Discussing potential side effects with medical professionals during treatment planning.
C. Nutritional Support:
1. Consulting with a registered dietitian for personalized nutrition plans.
2. Considering nutritional supplements if dietary intake is compromised.

Fatigue and Energy-Boosting Juices

Cancer patients often experience extreme fatigue as a result of both the disease itself and the treatments they undergo. This debilitating fatigue can affect their quality of life and make it challenging to maintain energy levels. One natural and nutritious way to combat this fatigue is by incorporating energy-boosting juices into their diet. In this comprehensive content, we will explore the causes of fatigue in cancer patients, the importance of nutrition, and provide a variety of juice recipes tailored to boost energy and overall well-being.

Section 1: Understanding Fatigue in Cancer Patients
1.1. Causes of Fatigue:
The impact of cancer on the body.
Side effects of cancer treatments (chemotherapy, radiation therapy, and surgery).

Emotional and psychological factors.

1.2. Consequences of Fatigue:

Reduced physical activity.

Impaired cognitive function.

Decreased quality of life.

Compromised immune system.

Section 2: The Role of Nutrition in Managing Fatigue

2.1. Nutritional Needs for Cancer Patients:

Maintaining a balanced diet.

Ensuring adequate calorie intake.

Protein, vitamins, and mineral requirements.

2.2. Benefits of Juices:

Easily digestible.

Provide essential nutrients.

Hydration and electrolyte balance.

Antioxidant properties.

Section 3: Energy-Boosting Juice Ingredients

3.1. Fruits:

High-energy fruits like bananas, oranges, and mangoes.

Berries rich in antioxidants (blueberries, strawberries).

3.2. Vegetables:

Leafy greens (spinach, kale) for iron and vitamins.

Carrots for beta-carotene.

3.3. Herbs and Spices:

Ginger for anti-inflammatory properties.

Mint for digestive support.

Turmeric for its potential anti-cancer properties.

3.4. Liquid Bases:

Coconut water for hydration and electrolytes.

Almond milk for added creaminess.

Section 4: Energy-Boosting Juice Recipes

4.1. Supercharged Green Smoothie:

Ingredients: Spinach, banana, almond milk, chia seeds, honey.

Benefits: High in vitamins, iron, and fiber.

4.2. Citrus Zest Booster:

Ingredients: Oranges, pineapple, ginger, mint.

Benefits: Immune-boosting and refreshing.

4.3. Berry Blast:

Ingredients: Mixed berries, yogurt, honey.

Benefits: Antioxidant-rich and protein-packed.

4.4. Golden Elixir:

Ingredients: Turmeric, carrot, orange, ginger.

Benefits: Anti-inflammatory and immune-boosting.

Section 5: Incorporating Juices into the Cancer Patient's Diet

5.1. Consultation with a Dietitian:

Individualized dietary plans.

5.2. Safety Measures:

Ensure hygiene during preparation.

Monitor for allergies or sensitivities.

5.3. Gradual Introduction:

Start with small servings.

Observe how the patient responds.

Maintaining a Healthy Weight

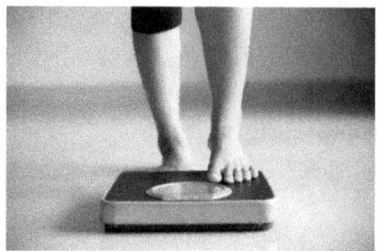

Maintaining a healthy weight as a cancer patient is crucial for your overall well-being and treatment outcomes. Cancer and its treatments can take a toll on your body, making it essential to focus on nutrition, physical activity, and emotional well-being to achieve and sustain a healthy weight. Here's a comprehensive guide to help you navigate this journey:

1. Consult with Your Healthcare Team:

Always start by consulting with your oncologist and a registered dietitian. They can provide personalized guidance based on your cancer type, treatment plan, and current health status.

2. Balanced Nutrition:

Aim for a balanced diet rich in fruits, vegetables, whole grains, lean proteins, and healthy fats.

Focus on nutrient-dense foods to support your immune system and aid in recovery.

Stay hydrated by drinking plenty of water, herbal teas, and clear broths to combat dehydration, a common side effect of cancer treatments.

3. Portion Control:

Be mindful of portion sizes to avoid overeating, which can lead to weight gain.

Use smaller plates and utensils to help with portion control.

4. **Manage Side Effects:**Cancer treatments often cause side effects like nausea, vomiting, and taste changes. Discuss these with your healthcare team, as they can affect your ability to maintain a healthy diet.

Consider trying smaller, more frequent meals to combat nausea.

5. **Include Protein:**

Protein is essential for tissue repair and immune function. Incorporate lean protein sources like chicken, fish, tofu, and legumes into your meals.

6. **Exercise Safely:**

Consult your healthcare team before starting any exercise program.

Incorporate gentle activities like walking, yoga, or swimming to maintain muscle mass, improve mood, and boost energy levels.

7. **Weight Monitoring:**

Regularly monitor your weight with guidance from your healthcare team. Sudden, unexplained weight loss or gain should be discussed with your healthcare provider.

8. **Emotional Support:**

Coping with cancer can be emotionally challenging. Seek support from a therapist, counselor, or support group to manage stress and emotional eating.

9. **Stay Informed:**

Stay informed about your cancer and treatment options. Knowledge can empower you to make informed decisions about your health and lifestyle.

10. **Avoid Fad Diets:**- Steer clear of extreme diets or supplements that promise quick fixes. These can be harmful and may interfere with your treatment.

11. **Set Realistic Goals:**

- Work with your healthcare team to set achievable goals for weight management. Small, gradual changes are often more sustainable.

12. **Family and Social Support:**

- Share your goals with your family and close friends, and seek their support in maintaining a healthy lifestyle.

13. **Manage Stress:**

- Incorporate stress-reduction techniques such as mindfulness, meditation, or deep breathing exercises into your daily routine to help manage emotional eating.

14. **Stay Positive:**

- Maintaining a positive outlook can have a significant impact on your overall well-being and your ability to adhere to a healthy lifestyle.

Remember that every cancer patient's journey is unique. Your healthcare team is your best resource for tailoring a plan that suits your specific needs and circumstances. By focusing on nutrition, physical activity, and emotional well-being, you can work towards maintaining a healthy weight and improving your quality of life during and after cancer treatment.

Hydration and Detoxification

Cancer is a complex group of diseases characterized by the uncontrolled growth and spread of abnormal cells. While the causes of cancer are multifactorial, there is growing interest in the role of hydration and detoxification in cancer prevention and management. This comprehensive guide explores the relationship between hydration, detoxification, and cancer, shedding light on how these factors can impact cancer risk, treatment, and overall well-being.

Section 1: Hydration and Cancer Risk

1.1 The Importance of Hydration:
Proper hydration is essential for overall health.

Dehydration can impair bodily functions and weaken the immune system, potentially increasing cancer risk.

1.2 Hydration and Cancer Prevention:

Staying hydrated may reduce the risk of certain cancers, such as bladder and colon cancer.

Adequate water intake helps the body flush out toxins and maintain healthy cell function.

Section 2: Detoxification and Cancer

2.1 Detoxification and Toxins:

Detoxification refers to the body's natural processes for eliminating harmful substances.

Exposure to environmental toxins, like pesticides and pollutants, can contribute to cancer development.

2.2 Detoxification Pathways:

The liver, kidneys, and lymphatic system play crucial roles in detoxification.

Proper nutrition and lifestyle choices can support these detox pathways.

Section 3: Hydration and Detoxification for Cancer Patients

3.1 Hydration during Cancer Treatment:

Cancer treatments, such as chemotherapy and radiation, can lead to dehydration.

Maintaining hydration is crucial to mitigate treatment side effects and support recovery.

3.2 Detoxification Support:

Some complementary therapies, like herbal remedies and dietary changes, claim to support detoxification during cancer treatment.

Consultation with healthcare professionals is essential to ensure safe practices.

Section 4: Debunking Detox Myths

4.1 Detox Diets and Cancer:

There is limited scientific evidence to support the efficacy of popular detox diets in preventing or curing cancer.

Extreme detox regimens can be harmful and should be approached with caution.

4.2 Promoting Healthful Detoxification:

Focus on a balanced diet rich in fruits, vegetables, and antioxidants to support the body's natural detoxification processes.

Lifestyle choices such as regular exercise, adequate sleep, and stress management are crucial for overall health.

Chapter6: Integrating Juicing into Your Cancer Journey

A cancer diagnosis can be overwhelming, and it often prompts individuals to explore complementary approaches to support their conventional treatment. One such approach is juicing, which involves extracting the liquid from fruits and vegetables. While juicing alone cannot cure cancer, it can be a valuable addition to your cancer journey by providing essential nutrients, hydration, and potential symptom relief.

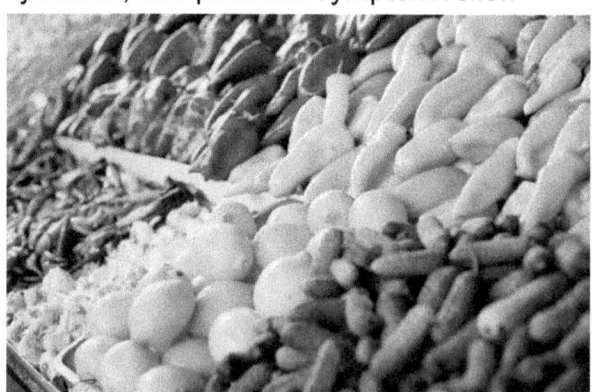

Nutrient-Rich Support:

Fruits and vegetables are packed with vitamins, minerals, and antioxidants that are crucial for overall health and immune function.

Juicing allows you to consume a variety of nutrients from different produce in an easily digestible form.

Hydration and Digestion:

Cancer treatments like chemotherapy can lead to dehydration and digestive issues. Fresh juices can help maintain hydration and soothe the digestive system.

Choosing hydrating ingredients like cucumber and watermelon can be especially beneficial.

Potential Symptom Management:

Certain juices may offer relief from common cancer-related symptoms such as nausea, fatigue, and inflammation.

Ginger and mint, for example, can ease nausea, while turmeric may help reduce inflammation.

Personalized Juicing Plans:

Consult with a healthcare professional or a nutritionist to create a customized juicing plan tailored to your specific cancer type, treatment, and dietary needs.

Ensure that your juice recipes align with your medical advice.

Freshness and Quality:

Use organic produce when possible to minimize exposure to pesticides and chemicals.

Invest in a quality juicer to retain maximum nutrients and flavors.

Moderation and Balance:

While juicing can be beneficial, it should not replace whole foods in your diet.

Balance your juicing regimen with a well-rounded diet that includes whole grains, lean proteins, and other essential food groups.

Safety Considerations:

Be cautious with high-sugar juices, as excess sugar can negatively impact your health.

Always consult your healthcare team before making significant dietary changes, especially if you're undergoing cancer treatment.

Emotional and Psychological Support:

Juicing can be a therapeutic and empowering aspect of your cancer journey, offering a sense of control and positivity.

Share this experience with loved ones to build a support network.

Conclusion:

Integrating juicing into your cancer journey can be a holistic way to enhance your nutrition, manage symptoms, and contribute to your overall well-being. However, it should be approached with careful consideration, in consultation with your healthcare team. When done mindfully and in conjunction with conventional treatments, juicing can be a valuable tool to support your path to recovery and improved quality of life.

Working with Healthcare Professionals

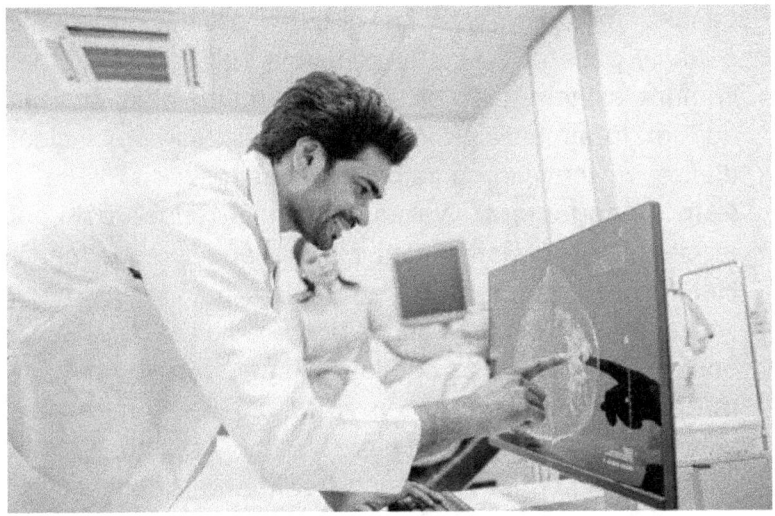

This collaborative journey encompasses physical, emotional, and informational aspects that are essential for cancer patients and their families.

Physical Benefits: Walking is a simple yet effective form of exercise that can help cancer patients manage symptoms and side effects of treatments like chemotherapy and radiation. It can improve cardiovascular health, reduce fatigue, and enhance overall fitness, leading to a better quality of life during and after treatment.

Emotional Support: Walking with healthcare professionals provides a supportive environment for patients to express their emotions and concerns. These professionals can offer counseling and guidance to help patients cope with the emotional challenges that cancer brings, such as anxiety, depression, and stress.

Nutritional Guidance: Nutrition plays a crucial role in cancer management. Healthcare professionals can educate patients on dietary choices that can boost their immune system, promote healing, and maintain strength during treatment. Walking discussions can include dietary advice tailored to individual needs.

Pain Management: Walking can help reduce pain and discomfort associated with cancer and its treatments. Healthcare professionals can monitor pain levels during walks and adjust medications or therapies accordingly to ensure patients are as comfortable as possible.

Information Sharing: Walking provides a relaxed setting for healthcare professionals to share vital information about cancer, treatment options, and potential side effects. Patients can ask questions and clarify doubts, leading to more informed decision-making.

Motivation and Accountability: Walking programs led by healthcare professionals offer patients motivation to stay active and adhere to their treatment plans. Knowing that someone is monitoring their progress can enhance compliance and overall well-being.

Peer Support: Walking groups often consist of patients facing similar challenges. Sharing experiences and insights can foster a sense of community and support. Healthcare professionals can facilitate these connections, allowing patients to learn from each other.

Monitoring Progress: Regular walks with healthcare professionals allow for the monitoring of a patient's physical and emotional progress. Any signs of deterioration or the emergence of new symptoms can be addressed promptly.

Long-term Wellness: Beyond cancer treatment, walking programs with healthcare professionals can help patients establish long-term wellness habits. This can include maintaining a healthy lifestyle to reduce the risk of cancer recurrence or managing the side effects of survivorship.

In conclusion, walking with healthcare professionals in the context of cancer care is a comprehensive approach that encompasses physical fitness, emotional support, education, and overall well-being. It promotes a collaborative journey towards better health and a higher quality of life for cancer patients.

Combining Juicing with Conventional Treatment

While conventional medical treatments like chemotherapy, radiation, and surgery remain essential in cancer management, there is a growing interest in complementary therapies to enhance overall well-being. One such approach is incorporating fresh fruit and vegetable juicing into the treatment regimen for cancer patients. This article explores the potential benefits, considerations, and precautions of combining juicing with conventional cancer treatments.

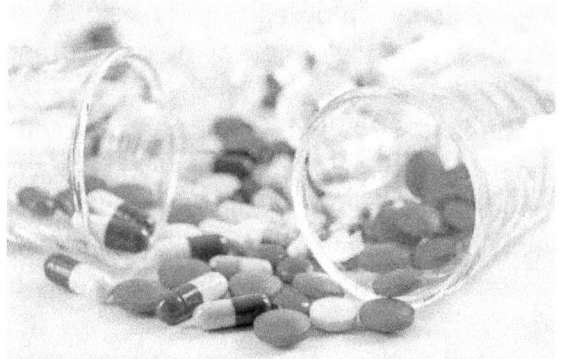

The Power of Juicing:

Juicing involves extracting the liquid content from fresh fruits and vegetables, providing a concentrated source of essential vitamins, minerals, and antioxidants. For cancer patients, these nutrients can play a crucial role in supporting overall health and aiding the body's natural defense mechanisms. Some potential benefits of juicing for cancer patients include:

Nutrient-Rich Diet: Cancer treatments can often cause appetite loss or digestive issues. Juicing provides a convenient way to ensure patients receive vital nutrients even when eating solid foods is challenging.

Hydration: Maintaining proper hydration is vital during cancer treatment. Fresh juices can help cancer patients stay hydrated while providing essential nutrients.

Antioxidant Support: Many fruits and vegetables are rich in antioxidants, which can help combat oxidative stress caused by cancer and its treatments.

Improved Digestion: Juicing can be easier to digest for patients experiencing nausea or gastrointestinal discomfort.

Considerations and Precautions:

While juicing can offer numerous benefits, it's essential to approach it with caution and in consultation with healthcare professionals:

Individualized Plans: Cancer patients should work with their oncologists or dietitians to create a personalized juicing plan that aligns with their specific medical needs and treatment protocols.

Avoid Sugary Juices: Some fruits can be high in natural sugars. Patients should prioritize vegetable-based juices and limit the consumption of sugary fruits to prevent blood sugar spikes.

Food Safety: Ensure that all fruits and vegetables used in juicing are thoroughly washed and safe to consume to minimize the risk of infections, especially for immunocompromised patients.

Potential Interactions: Certain fruits and vegetables may interact with medications or treatments. Discuss potential interactions with healthcare providers.

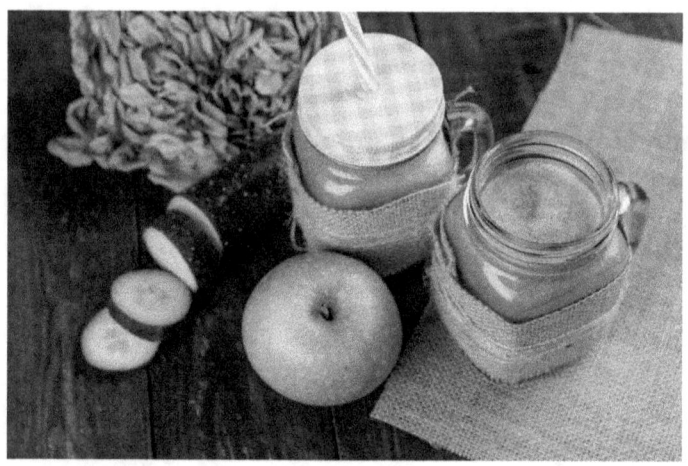

Conclusion:
Combining juicing with conventional cancer treatment is a holistic approach that aims to enhance the overall well-being of patients. When approached thoughtfully and in coordination with healthcare professionals, juicing can be a valuable addition to a cancer patient's diet. While it is not a standalone treatment for cancer, it can complement conventional therapies, support overall health, and improve the quality of life during the challenging journey of cancer treatment. Always consult with healthcare providers to ensure the safety and effectiveness of juicing as part of a cancer care plan.

Lifestyle and Dietary Changes

A cancer diagnosis is a life-altering event that often necessitates significant lifestyle and dietary changes to support the treatment process, manage side effects, and promote overall well-being. These changes play a crucial role in enhancing the quality of life and improving the chances of successful recovery. In this comprehensive text, we will explore the various aspects of lifestyle and dietary modifications for cancer patients.

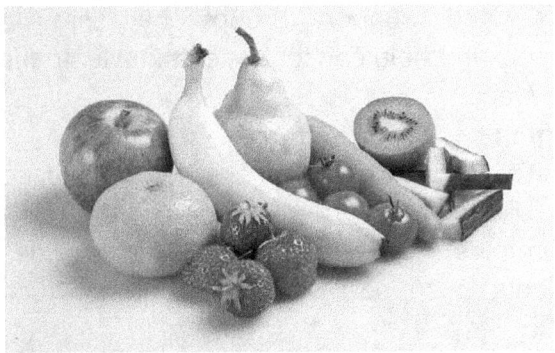

Lifestyle Changes:

Physical Activity: Maintaining a regular exercise routine can help cancer patients combat fatigue, improve mood, and enhance physical functioning. Consultation with a healthcare professional is essential to create a personalized exercise plan, considering the type and stage of cancer.

Stress Management: Cancer can be emotionally taxing. Engaging in stress-reduction techniques such as mindfulness meditation, yoga, or counseling can aid in coping with anxiety and depression.

Tobacco and Alcohol Cessation: Quitting smoking and limiting alcohol intake is imperative, as they are known risk factors for several types of cancer. Support groups and therapies are available to assist with addiction.

Rest and Sleep: Ensuring adequate rest and quality sleep is crucial for the body's healing process. Establishing a sleep routine and creating a comfortable sleep environment can be beneficial.

Social Support: Building a strong support network of family, friends, and support groups can provide emotional support and help cancer patients navigate the challenges they face.

Dietary Changes:

Balanced Diet: Cancer patients should aim for a well-balanced diet rich in fruits, vegetables, whole grains, lean proteins, and healthy fats. This provides essential nutrients to support the immune system and overall health.

Hydration: Staying adequately hydrated is vital, especially during cancer treatment. Drinking plenty of water can help manage side effects like nausea and fatigue.

Nutrient Density: Focus on nutrient-dense foods that provide vitamins, minerals, and antioxidants. These can help reduce inflammation and support the body's defenses.

Caloric Needs: Consult with a registered dietitian to determine your individual calorie and nutrient requirements. Some cancer treatments may affect appetite and digestion, and a tailored plan can address these issues.

Limit Processed Foods: Minimize the consumption of processed foods, sugary snacks, and high-fat items. These can contribute to weight gain and inflammation.

Special Diets: In some cases, specific diets like a low-fiber diet for digestive issues or a neutropenic diet to reduce infection risk may be recommended. Always follow medical advice regarding dietary restrictions.

Supplements: Discuss the use of supplements (e.g., vitamins, minerals) with your healthcare team. Taking supplements without guidance can sometimes be counterproductive.

Safe Food Handling: Chemotherapy and radiation therapy can weaken the immune system. Practicing safe food handling and avoiding raw or undercooked foods helps reduce the risk of foodborne illnesses.

Meal Timing: Eating smaller, more frequent meals throughout the day can help manage nausea and maintain energy levels.

It's crucial to remember that every cancer patient's journey is unique. Consultation with healthcare professionals, including oncologists, registered dietitians, and mental health experts, is essential to tailor these lifestyle and dietary changes to individual needs and treatment plans.

Chapter7: Success Stories and Testimonials

Meet Sarah, a resilient individual who confronted a daunting diagnosis: advanced stage breast cancer. Faced with the challenging road of treatments and therapies, she embarked on a transformative journey by incorporating natural fruits and vegetables into her daily diet to complement her medical care.

Sarah's Story:

In early 2020, Sarah received the life-changing news of her cancer diagnosis. Devastated but determined, she decided to explore complementary approaches to her conventional treatment plan. Sarah researched extensively and discovered the potential benefits of a plant-based diet rich in fruits and vegetables, renowned for their cancer-fighting properties

Testimonials:

Testimonial 1: Jennifer

Jennifer, a close friend of Sarah, witnessed her journey firsthand. "When Sarah decided to incorporate more fruits and vegetables into her diet, I was skeptical at first. But her commitment and optimism were inspiring.

Over time, I saw a remarkable change in her energy levels and overall well-being. It was as if the natural foods were empowering her body to fight back."

Testimonial 2: Dr. Patel, Oncologist

Dr. Patel, Sarah's oncologist, acknowledges the importance of nutrition in cancer care. "While I always emphasize the importance of medical treatments, I was supportive of Sarah's decision to improve her diet with natural foods. Fruits and vegetables contain antioxidants and nutrients that can aid the body in coping with the effects of cancer and its treatments."

Testimonial 3: Lisa, Sarah's Nutritionist

Lisa, a nutritionist specializing in oncology, played a vital role in Sarah's journey. "We worked closely to create a personalized dietary plan that included a variety of colorful fruits and vegetables. These foods not only provided essential nutrients but also helped manage some of the side effects of chemotherapy and radiation."

Testimonial 4: Sarah's Own Words

Sarah herself reflects on her journey: "Incorporating natural foods into my diet was a turning point in my battle against cancer. The fresh fruits and vegetables not only gave me physical strength but also boosted my spirits. They became a symbol of hope and vitality for me."

Over the course of her treatment, Sarah experienced a noticeable improvement in her health. While her journey included the conventional medical therapies recommended by her oncologist, she believes that the power of natural foods played a pivotal role in her healing process. Sarah is now an advocate for the benefits of incorporating fruits and vegetables into the diets of cancer patients, offering support and guidance to those facing similar challenges.

Sarah's success story and the testimonials of those who witnessed her transformation serve as a testament to the potential benefits of a diet rich in natural, cancer-fighting foods. It's essential to remember that while nutrition can be a valuable complement to medical treatments, it should always be discussed and coordinated with healthcare professionals to ensure it aligns with an individual's unique medical needs and treatment plants.

Real-Life Experiences of Cancer Survivors

Cancer survivors have diverse and inspiring stories to share. Many find strength and resilience in their journey. Some common themes in their experiences include:

Diagnosis: The shock and fear that come with a cancer diagnosis can be overwhelming. It's a pivotal moment that often leads to a search for the best treatment options.

Treatment: Survivors endure various treatments like surgery, chemotherapy, radiation therapy, and immunotherapy. These treatments can be physically and emotionally taxing.

Support: The support of family, friends, and healthcare providers is crucial. Survivors often speak about the importance of a strong support system in their recovery.

Coping: Coping strategies vary but may include meditation, counseling, or joining support groups to connect with others who've faced similar challenges.

Uncertainty: The fear of cancer recurrence is a common concern for survivors, leading them to adopt a "one day at a time" mindset.

Finding Purpose: Many survivors discover a renewed sense of purpose or a desire to give back through advocacy or volunteering in cancer-related causes.

Resilience: Overcoming cancer often highlights one's resilience and ability to adapt to life's challenges. These stories underscore the strength and determination of cancer survivors, offering hope and inspiration to others facing similar battles.

Inspiring Stories of Recovery Through Juicing

Name: Sarah
Background: Sarah was a vibrant and healthy woman in her mid-40s when she received the devastating news of her breast cancer diagnosis. Determined to fight the

disease with every tool available, she embarked on a challenging yet inspiring journey as a cancer survivor.

Diagnosis and Treatment: After her diagnosis, Sarah underwent a series of treatments including surgery, chemotherapy, and radiation therapy. While these treatments were crucial in her battle against cancer, they took a toll on her body, leaving her fatigued and often nauseous.

Discovering Juicing: During her treatment, Sarah researched alternative ways to support her body's healing process. She came across the concept of juicing, which involved extracting fresh juices from fruits and vegetables to provide essential nutrients. Intrigued by the potential benefits, she decided to incorporate juicing into her daily routine.

The Juicing Journey: Sarah started by investing in a high-quality juicer and began experimenting with various juice recipes. She learned which fruits and vegetables were rich in antioxidants, vitamins, and minerals that could boost her immune system and combat the side effects of her treatments.

Benefits of Juicing: Increased Energy: Sarah noticed a significant increase in her energy levels m as she started juicing regularly. This newfound vitality allowed her to cope better with the fatigue caused by chemotherapy.

Improved Digestion: Juicing helped soothe her digestive system, alleviating some of the nausea and digestive discomfort associated with chemotherapy.

Enhanced Nutrient Intake: By consuming a variety of fresh juices, Sarah ensured that her body received a wide range of nutrients, aiding in her overall well-being.

Weight Management: Juicing helped her maintain a healthy weight, which was essential for her recovery.

Mental Resilience: Preparing and enjoying fresh juices became a therapeutic and positive daily ritual for Sarah. It provided her with a sense of control and hope during her cancer journey.

Support System: Sarah's family and friends rallied around her, assisting with shopping for fresh produce, juicing, and even researching the best juice recipes for cancer patients. They joined her on her juicing journey, making it a bonding experience.

Recovery and Beyond: Sarah's determination, combined with her commitment to juicing, played a pivotal role in her recovery. Over time, her cancer went into remission, and she continued to prioritize her health through a balanced diet and regular exercise.

Inspiration: Sarah's journey served as an inspiration to others facing cancer. She shared her experiences and juice recipes through a blog and local support groups, helping fellow survivors explore the benefits of juicing.

Conclusion: Sarah's story demonstrates the potential benefits of incorporating juicing into the cancer survivor experience. While it's essential to consult with medical professionals and use juicing as a complementary approach to traditional cancer treatments, her journey exemplifies the positive impact that a holistic approach to health can have on the road to recovery.

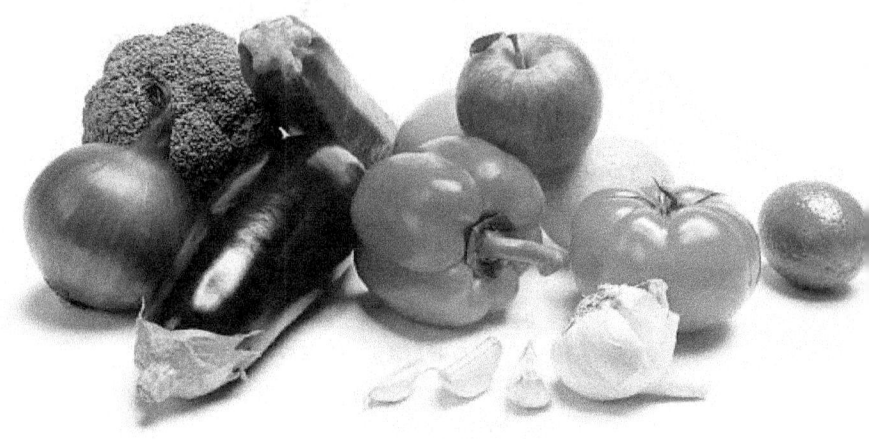

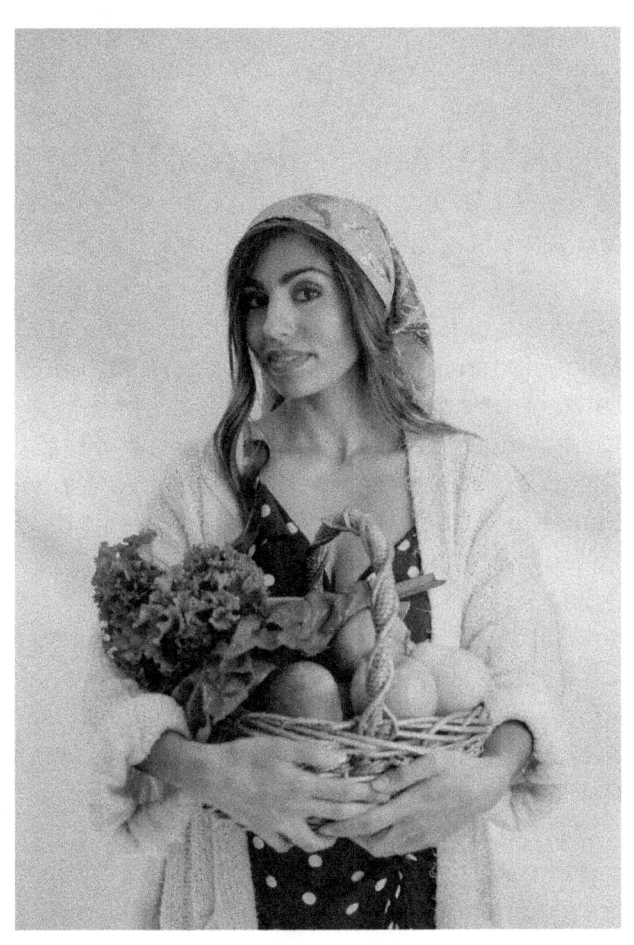

Chapter8: Beyond Cancer

Cancer is a formidable adversary, affecting millions of lives worldwide. It can be a devastating diagnosis, but it's essential to remember that life extends beyond cancer. In this comprehensive content, we will explore the many facets of life beyond cancer, focusing on hope, resilience, and the incredible stories of survivors who have triumphed over this disease.

Section 1: The Power of Hope

The Mental Battle: Cancer often comes with a mental and emotional toll. Maintaining hope is crucial for healing and recovery.

Medical Advances: Advancements in cancer treatment provide newfound hope for patients, increasing survival rates and quality of life.

Support Systems: Friends, family, and support groups offer emotional support, reinforcing the idea that life is worth fighting for.

Section 2: Resilience in the Face of Adversity

Overcoming Challenges: Cancer patients display remarkable resilience in battling the physical and emotional challenges associated with their diagnosis.

. **Survivor Stories:** Share inspiring stories of cancer survivors who have not only beaten the odds but emerged stronger and more resilient.

. **Coping Mechanisms:** Explore various coping strategies that help patients and survivors navigate the difficult journey, from mindfulness to creative expression.

Section 3: Life Beyond Cancer

Regaining Control: After treatment, individuals often regain a sense of control over their lives, allowing them to pursue their dreams and passions.

Healthy Living: Emphasize the importance of a healthy lifestyle post-cancer, including exercise, nutrition, and regular check-ups.

. **Redefining Priorities:** Many survivors discover a renewed sense of purpose, reevaluating their life goals and priorities.

Section 4: Supporting the Journey

Medical Professionals: Recognize the dedication of healthcare providers who play a crucial role in guiding patients through their cancer journey.

Caregivers: Highlight the invaluable support provided by caregivers who stand by their loved ones during the most challenging times.

. **Research and Advocacy:** Discuss the significance of cancer research and advocacy in improving treatment options and raising awareness.

Conclusion:
Cancer is a formidable adversary, but it is not the end of life's journey. Hope, resilience, and the support of a loving community can help individuals not only survive

but thrive beyond cancer. By sharing stories of triumph and emphasizing the importance of a holistic approach to healing, we can inspire those affected by cancer to embrace life beyond this diagnosis, knowing that a brighter future awaits them.

Maintaining a Healthy Lifestyle Post-Cancer

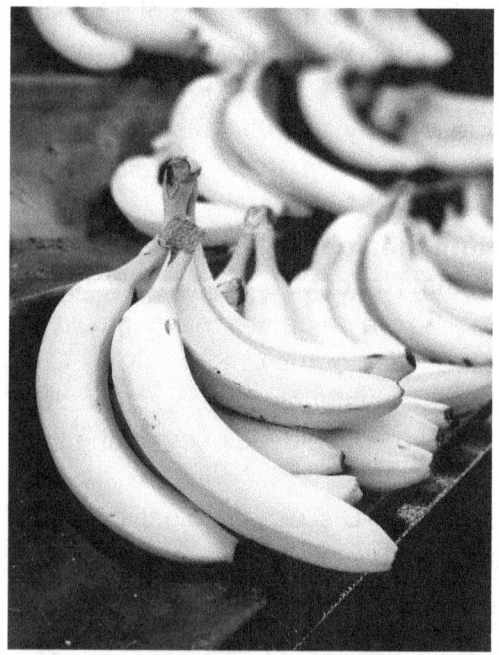

Maintaining a healthy lifestyle post-cancer is crucial for overall well-being. Here are some key aspects to focus on:

Diet: Eat a balanced diet rich in fruits, vegetables, whole grains, lean proteins, and low-fat dairy. Limit processed foods, sugary drinks, and excessive red meat consumption.

Physical activity: Establish time for regular exercise, aiming towards at least two hours of aerobic activity of a moderate level per week. For advice on what is suitable and safe for you, speak with your healthcare provider. Stay Hydrated: Drink plenty of water to stay properly hydrated. Limit or avoid alcohol, as it can increase the risk of certain cancers.

Regular Check-Ups: Continue with follow-up appointments and screenings as recommended by your healthcare team to monitor for recurrence or new health issues.

Manage Stress: Practice stress-reduction techniques like meditation, yoga, or mindfulness to help cope with the emotional impact of cancer.

Get Adequate Sleep: Aim for 7-9 hours of quality sleep per night to support your body's healing and overall health.

Quit Smoking: The best thing you could do for your health is to stop smoking if you currently do so. To help anyone quit, look for help and support.

Limit Sun Exposure: Protect your skin from the sun to reduce the risk of skin cancer by wearing sunscreen, protective clothing, and avoiding peak sunlight hours.

Social Support: Connect with friends and family for emotional support. Consider joining a cancer support group to share experiences and strategies.

Stay Informed: Stay informed about the latest research on cancer survivorship and treatment options. Knowledge is empowering.

Remember that your specific needs may vary depending on the type of cancer and treatment you received. Always consult with your healthcare team for personalized advice and guidance tailored to your situation.

Preventative Juicing for a Cancer-Free Future

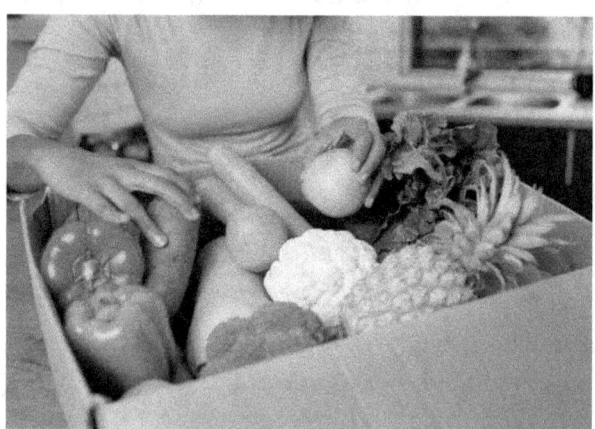

While a healthy diet rich in fruits and vegetables can contribute to overall well-being, it's essential to approach health claims about preventing cancer with caution. There is no specific "preventative juicing" regimen that guarantees a cancer-free future. Cancer is a complex disease influenced by various factors, including genetics, lifestyle, and environmental exposures.

To reduce your risk of cancer, consider these general guidelines:

Eat a Balanced Diet: Consume a variety of fruits, vegetables, whole grains, lean proteins, and healthy fats.

Maintain a Healthy Weight: Obesity is linked to an increased risk of certain cancers. Maintain a healthy body weight through diet and exercise.

Limit Processed Foods: Minimize your intake of processed meats, sugary drinks, and highly processed foods, which may be associated with cancer risk.

Stay Active: Regular physical activity can help lower your risk of cancer and improve overall health.

Avoid Smoking and Limit Alcohol: Smoking is a leading cause of cancer, and excessive alcohol consumption is also associated with increased cancer risk.

Protect Against UV Radiation: Use sunscreen and protective clothing to reduce your risk of skin cancer.

Get Screened: Follow recommended cancer screening guidelines for your age and risk factors.

Know Your Family History: Some cancers have a hereditary component, so understanding your family's medical history is important.

While juicing can be a part of a healthy diet, it's crucial not to rely solely on it as a cancer prevention strategy. A well-rounded, balanced diet, coupled with a healthy lifestyle, is the best approach to reducing your risk of cancer and promoting overall health. Consult with a healthcare professional for personalized advice based on your individual health needs and risk factors.

Conclusion

In conclusion, juicing for cancer is a topic that has garnered attention due to its potential health benefits. While some studies suggest that consuming fresh fruit and vegetable juices may provide nutrients and antioxidants that could support overall health and potentially aid in cancer prevention, it's important to note that juicing should not be considered a sole or primary treatment for cancer.

A balanced diet, rich in a variety of fruits, vegetables, and other whole foods, combined with medical treatments prescribed by healthcare professionals, remains the standard approach for managing cancer. Juicing can be a complementary part of a healthy lifestyle, but individuals with cancer should consult with their healthcare team before making significant dietary changes to ensure they are making choices that align with their specific needs and treatment plan.

Ultimately, while juicing can be a flavorful and nutritious addition to one's diet, it should be viewed as a part of an overall strategy for maintaining health and well-being, rather than a standalone solution for cancer prevention or treatment. Always seek guidance from healthcare professionals for personalized advice when dealing with cancer or any serious medical condition.

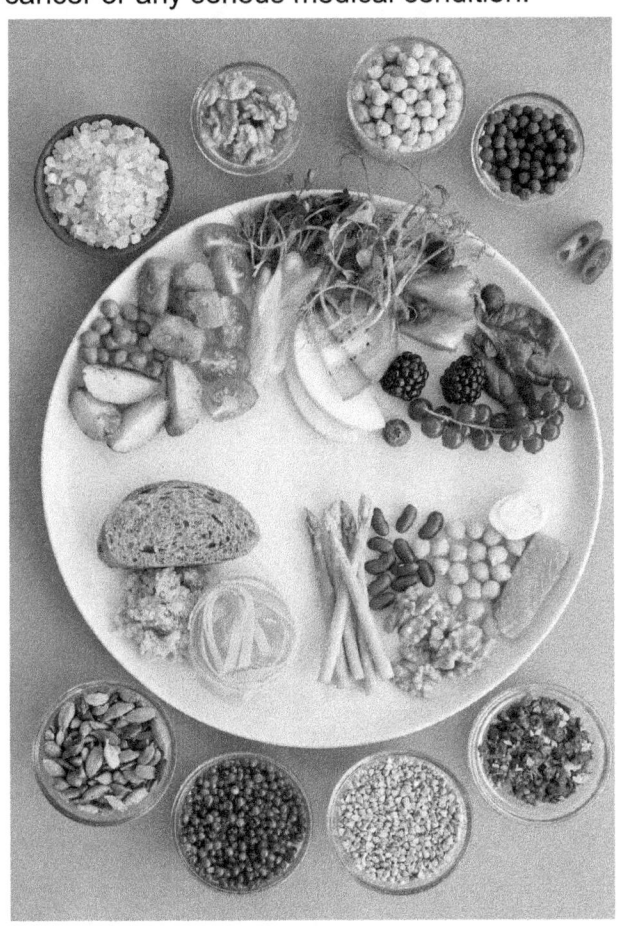

www.ingramcontent.com/pod-product-compliance
Lightning Source LLC
Chambersburg PA
CBHW072309290526
45794CB00002B/593